Study Guide to Accompany

Surgical Technology for the Surgical Technologist: A Positive Care Approach

The Association of Surgical Technologists, Inc.

Second Edition

Study Guide to Accompany

Surgical Technology for the Surgical Technologist: A Positive Care Approach

The Association of Surgical Technologists, Inc.

Second Edition

Teri L. Junge, CST/CFA

Surgical Technology Program Director
San Joaquin Valley College, Fresno, CA

THOMSON

DELMAR LEARNING   Australia Canada Mexico Singapore Spain United Kingdom United States

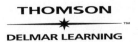

THOMSON

DELMAR LEARNING

Study Guide to Accompany Surgical Technology for the Surgical Technologist, Second Edition
The Association of Surgical Technologists
Teri L. Junge, CST/CFA

Vice President, Health Care Business Unit:
William Brottmilter

Editorial Director:
Cathy L. Esperti

Acquisitions Editor:
Rhonda Dearborn

Developmental Editor:
Marjorie A. Bruce

Marketing Director:
Jennifer McAvey

Marketing Coordinator:
Jill Osterhout

Editorial Assistant:
Natalie Wager

Art/Design Specialist:
Connie Lundberg-Watkins

Production Coordinator:
Bridget Lulay

Project Editor:
Jim Zayicek

Library of Congress Cataloging-in-Publication Data

ISBN 1-4018-3849-9

Notice to the Reader:
Publisher does not warrant or guarantee any of the products described herein or perform any independent analysis in connection with any of the product information contained herein. Publisher does not assume, and expressly disclaims, any obligation to obtain and include information other than that provided to it by the manufacturer.

The reader is expressly warned to consider and adopt all safety precautions that might be indicated by the activities described herein and to avoid all potential hazards. By following the instructions contained herein, the reader willingly assumes all risks in connection with such instructions.

The publisher makes no representations or warranties of any kind, including but not limited to, the warranties of fitness for particular purpose or merchantability, nor are any such representations implied with respect to the material set forth herein, and the publisher takes no responsibility with respect to such material. The publisher shall not be liable for any special, consequential, or exemplary damages resulting, in whole or part, from the reader's use of, or reliance upon, this material.

Contents

SKILL ASSESSMENT LIST AND LOCATOR

Skill Assessment (Name and Number)

Preface

TO THE SURGICAL TECHNOLOGY STUDENT

The textbook *Surgical Technology for the Surgical Technologist:A Positive Care Approach,* second edition defines the cognitive model necessary for the surgical technologist to function effectively and provides an innovative approach for learning the role of the surgical technologist while focusing on the knowledge and skills that will be required. This model leads the way for the surgical technology student to remember the pertinent information using the predictive model: *A Positive Care Approach.* Because the text was written by surgical technologists and surgical technology educators, the needs of the student have been considered throughout the process. The graduate of a CAAHEP (Commission on Accreditation of Allied Health Education Programs) accredited surgical technology program will meet the eligibility requirements of the LCC-ST (Liaison Council on Certification for the Surgical Technologist) to sit for the national certifying examination for the surgical technologist.

The basic steps of the cognitive process for the surgical technologist are defined by Bob Caruthers, CST, PhD, former Deputy Director, Association of Surgical Technologists.

The surgical technologist:

- has a mental image of normal anatomy
- makes a mental comparison of the idealized anatomy with the actual anatomy of a specific patient
- knows an idealized operative procedure used to correct the pathologic condition
- makes a mental comparison of the idealized procedure with the actual procedure being performed
- allows for a particular surgeon's variations to the idealized procedure
- allows for variances in anatomy, pathology, and surgeons' responses to the variances
- predicts and prepares to meet the needs of the surgeon and surgical patient prior to verbalization of the need

To facilitate the learning process, *Surgical Technology for the Surgical Technologist: A Positive Care Approach* has been divided into two major sections. These divisions correspond to *A Positive Care Approach* and are represented by the A POSitive and CARE acronyms. The first 12 chapters are related to the CARE acronym. The CARE division itself is divided into two sections: (1) Introduction to Surgical Technology, and (2) Principles and Practice of Surgical Technology. The last 12 chapters relate to the A POSitive acronym; a brief introduction to diagnostics is followed by chapters focusing on operative procedures for various surgical specialties.

What is the *A Positive Care Approach?* It is a systematic approach to surgical problem solving focused on the ability of the surgical technologist to predict the needs of the surgeon and patient. The *A Positive Care Approach* uses two simple memory tools for systematic problem solving.

The CARE division will establish a broad context in which the instructor will help the student place the more specific technical information that dominates surgical technology. Introductory and foundational information is learned using the CARE approach, which is intended to serve as a reminder to the surgical technologist that all activities affect the care given to the patient. The student should be aware that the highly variable topics of the first 12, or non-procedural, chapters of the text do not allow a simple one-to-one correlation of the CARE memory tool, rather, it is a conceptual tool intended to help organize the information:

C Care directed toward the patient and/or surgical team

A Aseptic principles and practice of sterile technique

R Role of the surgical technologist

E Environmental awareness and concern

The A POSitive division relates directly to the final 12, or procedural, chapters with CARE as the underlying theme. The surgical procedures are presented by surgical specialty using the illustrative procedure format. The illustrative procedure format is based on the concept that one procedure can highlight several important steps that are repeated in related procedures. Rather than presenting many procedures with brief outlines of the steps, fewer procedures are presented in greater detail, thus allowing the surgical technologist to predict the necessary preparation and action to be taken. The A POSitive approach does allow the one-to-one correlation of the procedural chapter objectives and should be used to reinforce every surgical procedure encountered by the student:

A Anatomy

P Pathology

O Operative Procedure

S Specific Variations

In this Study Guide, we will provide you with learning concepts and tools and a way to use them to enhance your education.

The authors of **Surgical Technology for the Surgical Technologist: A Positive Care Approach,** second edition, wish you success in your endeavor to become a Certified Surgical Technologist (CST)!

Orientation to Surgical Technology

CHAPTER 1

OBJECTIVES

After studying this chapter, the reader should be able to:

C 1. Identify and demonstrate principles of communication in the surgical setting.

A 2. (No objectives focused on asepsis in this chapter; however, the student should demonstrate an awareness that the principles of asepsis are a vital component of the surgical technologist's role in surgical patient care.)

R 3. Trace the historical development of surgery and surgical technology.

4. Identify members of the surgical team and their roles.

5. Identify the various roles of the surgical technologist.

6. Identify and interpret a job description for the surgical technologist.

E 7. Identify different types of health care facilities.

8. Describe a typical hospital organizational structure.

9. Identify hospital departments and their relationship to surgical services.

■ Select Key Terms

Define the following:

1. acronym _____

_____

2. ambulatory surgical facility_____

_____

3. ARC-ST _____

_____

4. AST _____

_____

5. circulator_____

_____

6. competency _____

_____

7. Core Curriculum _____

_____

8. DO_____

_____

9. elective _____

_____

10. emergent_____

_____

11. HMO _____

_____

12. intraoperative_____

_____

13. JCAHO _____

_____

14. LCC-ST _____

_____

15. optional _____

_____

16. Pasteur _____

_____

17. postoperative _____

_____

18. preceptor _____

_____

19. preoperative_____

_____

20. professional _____

_____

21. proprietary _____

_____

22. STSR _____

_____

23. urgent _____

_____

24. Vesalius_____

_____

■ Case Studies

□ CASE STUDY 1

Rodrigo is a 57-year-old male who was admitted to the emergency department (ED) following a motor vehicle accident. Rodrigo was driving a delivery van that was struck head-on by another vehicle. Rodrigo has severe injuries to both lower extremities: (1) closed femur fracture of the left leg and (2) open fracture of the right tibia and fibula with near amputation. A chest tube was inserted upon arrival in the ED. Rodrigo is neurologically intact. He is now scheduled for surgery on his legs.

1. This case represents what category of surgical intervention? _____

   _____

   _____

   _____

   _____

2. What is the difference between emergent and urgent surgical intervention? _____

   _____

   _____

   _____

   _____

3. What is elective surgery? _____

   _____

   _____

   _____

   _____

4. Is elective surgical intervention the same thing as "minor" surgery? _____

   _____

   _____

   _____

   _____

☐ CASE STUDY 2

Kathleen is a 15-year-old female who has been admitted to the hospital for surgery to correct a condition called scoliosis, an abnormal lateral curvature of the spine. This surgical intervention requires a lengthy incision and dissection of spinal muscles. It runs the risk of considerable blood loss and damage to spinal nerves. Distraction rods are placed to help straighten the spine, and bone grafting is required.

1. Intraoperative X-rays are required. Who would perform these, and what department of the hospital would employ them? _____

_____

_____

_____

2. Blood loss may be countered by filtering the patient's blood and returning it to her. Who would perform this activity? _____

_____

_____

_____

3. Patients undergoing spinal surgery are often monitored for changes in electrical conduction to the lower extremities. Who would perform this task? _____

_____

_____

_____

4. To whom would blood samples be taken in order to check the hematocrit and hemoglobin counts during the operative procedure? _____

_____

_____

_____

5. An upper body cast may be applied several days postoperatively. Who would assist the surgeon in this task?

_____

_____

_____

☐

CHAPTER 3

The Surgical Patient

OBJECTIVES

After studying this chapter, the reader should be able to:

C   1. Assess the patient's response to illness and hospitalization.

A   2. Demonstrate awareness that all surgical patients have the right to the highest standards and practices in asepsis.

R   3. Distinguish and assess the physical, spiritual, and psychological needs of a patient.

E   4. Distinguish and assess cultural and religious influences on the surgical patient.

■ Select Key Terms

Define the following:

1. Maslow's hierarchy of needs _____

2. patient _____

3. ~~vsical~~ need _____

4. psychological need _____

5. social need _____

6. spiritual need _____

■ Case Studies

□ CASE STUDY 1

Myrtle is scheduled for a total hip arthroplasty in about half an hour. She is in the preoperative holding area and has just expressed to her nurse a fear that she will not survive the procedure. Myrtle has asked to speak with the chaplain.

1. What type of need is Myrtle expressing? _____

   _____

   _____

   _____

   _____

2. Should her premonition be taken seriously? _____

   _____

   _____

   _____

3. With the procedure scheduled to take place shortly, will time allow the chaplain to be called? _____

   _____

   _____

   _____

   _____

☐ CASE STUDY 2

The circulator has just come to the preoperative holding area to pick up 18-month-old Henry to take him to the operating room for his ear surgery. Henry took one look at the circulator and began screaming and clinging to his mother.

1. Use the life tasks approach to determine if Henry's behavior is appropriate for his age group. _____

   _____

   _____

   _____

   _____

2. Using Maslow's hierarchy of needs, which of Henry's needs may not be met when he is taken from his mother by the circulator to go to the operating room? _____

   _____

   _____

   _____

   _____

3. What can be done to make the transition from being in his mother's care to being in the care of the circulator a smooth one for Henry? _____

   _____

   _____

   _____

   _____

☐

CHAPTER 4

Special Populations

OBJECTIVES

After studying this chapter, the reader should be able to:

C 1. Compare and contrast the surgical care considerations for pediatric patients and patients who are obese, diabetic, pregnant, immunocompromised, disabled, geriatric, or experiencing trauma.

2. Describe the unique physical and psychological need of each special population.

A 3. Compare and contrast the intraoperative considerations for pediatric patients and patients who are obese, diabetic, immunocompromised, geriatric, or traumatized that relate to postoperative wound healing.

R 4. Evaluate the role of the surgical technologist for the surgical care of each special population.

E 5. Assess the ethical commitment that is required of surgical technologists as it relates to special populations care.

6. Describe the general needs associated with special populations of surgical patients.

■ Select Key Terms

Define the following:

1. arterial blood gases (ABGs) _____

   _____

2. autoimmune diseases _____

   _____

3. central venous catheter_____

   _____

4. diabetes mellitus _____

   _____

5. enterocolitis _____

   _____

6. golden hour _____

   _____

7. human immunodeficiency virus (HIV) _____

   _____

8. hypothermia_____

   _____

9. immunocompetence _____

   _____

10. intra-arterial measurement _____

    _____

11. Kaposi's sarcoma _____

    _____

12. kinematics _____

    _____

13. penetrating trauma _____

    _____

14. pneumothorax _____

    _____

15. Revised Trauma Score_____

    _____

16. septic shock _____

    _____

17. splenectomy_____

    _____

18. splenomegaly_____

    _____

19. torticollis_____

    _____

20. urine output _____

    _____

21. venous compression device_____

    _____

■ Case Studies

☐ CASE STUDY 1

Seven-year-old Alexandra lost control of her scooter as she was riding down her sloped driveway. She inadvertently rode into the street and was hit by a car. She was not wearing a helmet.

1. What is the first priority of the emergency team that arrives at the scene to assist Alexandra? _____

   _____

   _____

   _____

   _____

2. The emergency team suspects that Alexandra may have sustained a neck injury during the accident. What should be done to protect the spinal cord?_____

   _____

   _____

   _____

3. Alexandra appears to be going into hypovolemic shock. What step(s) should be taken to prevent the hypovolemia from becoming severe?_____

   _____

   _____

   _____

   _____

   ☐

☐ CASE STUDY 2

Baby boy Daniels' birth was traumatic. He has suffered a bone fracture and the left side of his face appears to droop.

1. What is the most common type of bone fracture that occurs during traumatic birth? _____

    _____

    _____

    _____

    _____

2. What is most likely causing the neonate's face to droop? _____

    _____

    _____

    _____

    _____

3. Is the facial droop expected to resolve? If so, how soon? _____

    _____

    _____

    _____

    _____

    ☐

CHAPTER 6

Biomedical Science

OBJECTIVES

After studying this chapter, the reader should be able to:

C
1. Identify basic components of a computer system.
2. Describe electrical safety precautions.
3. Define terms related to physics.
4. Describe the basic concepts of robotics.

A
5. (No objectives focused on asepsis in this chapter; however, the practice of sterile technique will be necessary when using related equipment in the OR.)

R
6. Perform basic word processing, Internet, and e-mail functions.
7. Apply computer knowledge to safe patient care.
8. Describe the geometrical concepts of robotics and the mechanisms of the robotic system.

E
9. Describe the basic principles of electricity and their application in the OR.
10. Apply the principles of robotics to safe patient care practices in the OR.
11. Apply the principles of physics to safe patient care practices in the OR.

■ Select Key Terms

Define the following:

1. active electrode _____ _____

2. Cartesian coordinate geomet___ _____

3. central processing ___ (CPU) _____

4. circuit ____ _____

5. degree of freedom _____

___ dispersive (inactive) electrode _____

7. electrons _____

8. font _____

9. free electrons _____

10. generator _____

11. ground wire _____

12. hydraulic pressure _____

13. inertia _____

14. infrared waves _____

15. insulator _____

16. load _____

17. mass _____

18. modem _____

19. monitor _____

20. mouse _____

21. neutrons _____

22. periodic table _____

23. plasma _____

24. power _____

25. pressure _____

26. protons _____

27. quarks _____

28. refraction _____

29. resistance _____

30. switch _____

31. volume _____

32. weight _____   33. X-rays _____

_____   _____

■ Case Studies

☐ CASE STUDY 1

Norman is a surgical technologist who is circulating during a hip nailing. During the surgical procedure, the surgeon asks to see the patient's X-rays and blood test results since hepatitis B may be involved. Norman is going to use the computer in the operating room to send an e-mail requesting that the Radiology Department's unit secretary immediately bring over the patient's X-rays. He will send another e-mail to the laboratory technologist requesting that the blood test results be e-mailed to him in the OR.

1. Which icon will Norman use to create a new e-mail message? Where is the icon located and what does it look like? _____

_____

_____

_____

_____

2. Norman wants to emphasize the patient's name and facility identification number. Briefly describe two ways to create emphasis using word processing functions. _____

_____

_____

_____

_____

3. Norman wants to ensure that the individual at the surgery department control desk sees the e-mail (so that he or she will know which OR to deliver the X-rays to when they arrive), but that individual does not need to reply. What function would Norman use? _____

_____

_____

_____

_____

(continues)

☐ CASE STUDY 1 (*continued*)

4. Norman recently visited the CDC website and noticed an update on hepatitis B. List three ways that he can find that site again. _____

    _____

    _____

    _____

    _____

    ☐

☐ CASE STUDY 2

A female patient is brought to the operating room for a right oophorectomy. The surgeon is planning to use the AESOP robotic system to perform the surgical procedure. The STSR is responsible for setting up the robotic manipulator before the patient enters the OR.

1. On which side of the operating table should the manipulator be placed? _____

    _____

    _____

    _____

    _____

2. For optimal positioning of the endoscope, should the manipulator be placed at the head, midsection, or foot of the operating table? _____

    _____

    _____

    _____

    _____

3. When positioning the manipulator, what additional mechanism can be used to create more clearance between the elbow of the manipulator and the patient? _____

    _____

    _____

    _____

    _____

    ☐

CHAPTER 7

Asepsis and Sterile Technique

OBJECTIVES

After studying this chapter, the reader should be able to:

C 1. Discuss the relationship between the principles of asepsis and practice of sterile technique and surgical patient care.

2. Define and discuss the concept of surgical conscience.

A 3. Discuss the principles of asepsis.

4. Define the terms related to asepsis.

5. Discuss the sterile practices related to the principles of asepsis.

6. Identify the principles and procedures related to disinfection and sterilization.

R 7. Demonstrate competency related to the practice of sterile technique.

8. Demonstrate competency in the procedures related to disinfection and sterilization.

E 9. Discuss the surgical environment and the application of the principles of asepsis to the environment.

■ Select Key Terms

Define the following:

1. asepsis _____

_____

2. autoclave _____

_____

3. bioburden _____

_____

4. biological indicator _____

_____

5. Bowie-Dick test _____

_____

6. chelation _____

_____

7. chemical indicator _____

_____

8. colonization _____

_____

9. contaminated _____

_____

10. emulsification _____

_____

11. endoscope _____

_____

12. event-related sterility _____

_____

13. flash sterilization _____

_____

14. immersion _____

_____

15. integrity _____

_____

16. intermediate-level disinfection _____

_____

17. Julian date _____

_____

18. Lister _____

_____

19. lumen _____

_____

20. pathogen _____

_____

21. permeability _____

_____

22. sterile field _____

_____

23. sterile technique _____

_____

24. sterilization _____

_____

25. surgical conscience _____

_____

26. ultrasonic washer _____

_____

Case Studies

CASE STUDY 1

Brittney telephones her physician to report that she is experiencing a fever of 101°F seven days following her laparoscopic tubal ligation. She also states that she is experiencing urinary frequency and burning during urination. The physician suspects that Brittney may be suffering from a urinary tract infection be- cause of the catheter that was used to empty her blad- der during the surgical procedure. The physician has asked Brittney to schedule an appointment later in the day so that he may examine her and obtain a "clean catch" urine sample.

1. Would Brittney's infection be considered a surgical site infection (SSI)? If not, what type of infection is it?

   _____

   _____

   _____

   _____

2. What is the most likely reason that Brittney is suffering from an infection?

   _____

   _____

   _____

   _____

CASE STUDY 2

Ned is preparing the operating room for an emer- gency procedure. He is rushing because he knows that the patient will soon be brought into the room and he may not have time to complete his prepara- tions. Ned is opening the final item; just as he is about to place the item on the back table, he notices a small hole in the wrapper.

1. What moral/ethical concept will Ned use to make the "right" decision?

   _____

   _____

   _____

   _____

(continues)

☐ CASE STUDY 2 (*continued*)

2. What are Ned's options, and what is the best choice?

    _____

    _____

    _____

    _____

3. If Ned makes the wrong choice, what possible impact could this have on the patient?

    _____

    _____

    _____

    _____

    ☐

Basic Handwash

Student Name _____ Date _____

Instructor _____

Procedural Step	Adequate	Needs Review
1. Student is able to state purpose of handwash		
2. Student is able to state circumstances when a handwash is necessary		
3. Equipment and supplies are assembled		
4. Jewelry removed		
5. Turn on faucet		
6. Inspect hands and wrists		
7. Wet hands and wrists		
8. Apply soap		
9. Lather		
10. Interlace fingers		
11. Use nail cleaner/brush (if necessary)		
12. Handwash is of appropriate duration		
13. All surfaces cleaned		
14. Rinse		
15. Turn off water		
16. Dry		
17. Discard towel(s)		

Comments _____

_____

_____

_____

Packaging Technique – Wrap
(Envelope Fold)

Student Name _____ Date _____

Instructor _____

Procedural Step	Adequate	Needs Review
1. Student is able to state purpose for envelope-style wrap		
2. Appropriate attire		
3. Wash hands (Standard Precautions)		
4. Equipment and supplies assembled		
5. Orient wrap material on suitable surface		
6. Place item to be wrapped on wrapper		
7. Insert internal indicator		
8. Fold first flap		
9. Fold second (left) flap		
10. Fold third (right) flap		
11. Fold fourth flap		
12. Apply second wrapper (if necessary)		
13. Secure final flap		
14. Label for processing		
15. Place in designated area		
16. Proceed with other tasks		

Comments _____

_____

_____

_____

Packaging Technique – Wrap
(Square Fold)

Student Name _____ Date _____

Instructor _____

Procedural Step	Adequate	Needs Review
1. Student is able to state purpose for square-style wrap		
2. Appropriate attire		
3. Wash hands (Standard Precautions)		
4. Equipment and supplies assembled		
5. Orient wrap material on suitable surface		
6. Place item to be wrapped on wrapper		
7. Insert internal indicator		
8. Fold first flap		
9. Fold second flap		
10. Fold third flap		
11. Fold final flap		
12. Apply second wrapper (if necessary)		
13. Secure final flap		
14. Label for processing		
15. Place in designated area		
16. Proceed with other tasks		

Comments _____

_____

_____

_____

Packaging Technique – Peel Pack

Student Name _____ Date _____

Instructor _____

Procedural Step	Adequate	Needs Review
1. Student is able to state purpose for peel pack-style package		
2. Appropriate attire		
3. Wash hands (Standard Precautions)		
4. Equipment and supplies assembled		
5. Place item(s) in pouch		
6. Seal pouch		
7. Double package (if necessary)		
8. Label for processing		
9. Place in designated area		
10. Proceed with other tasks		

Comments _____

_____

_____

_____

Packaging Technique – Container System

Student Name _____ Date _____

Instructor _____

Procedural Step	Adequate	Needs Review
1. Student is able to state purpose for container-style package		
2. Appropriate attire		
3. Wash hands (Standard Precautions)		
4. Equipment and supplies assembled		
5. Prepare container		
6. Place instrument set in basket		
7. Place basket in container		
8. Place lid and seal		
9. Label for processing		
10. Place in designated area		
11. Proceed with other tasks		

Comments _____

_____

_____

_____

CHAPTER 8

General Patient Care and Safety

OBJECTIVES

After studying this chapter, the reader should be able to:

C 1. Demonstrate an understanding of the process used to obtain an informed consent for a surgical procedure or treatment.

2. Describe preoperative routines.

3. Identify, describe, and demonstrate the principles of transportation of the surgical patient.

4. Discuss, demonstrate, and apply the principles of surgical positioning.

5. Understand the methods of preparation of the operative site for surgery.

6. Describe the application of thermoregulatory devices.

7. Explain the principles and demonstrate the taking and recording of vital signs.

8. Explain the principles of urinary catheterization and demonstrate the procedure.

A 9. Describe how the principles of operative site preparation and urinary catheterization are related both to patient care and to the principles of asepsis.

R 10. Discuss methods of hemostasis and blood replacement and demonstrate the preparation and use of appropriate agents or devices.

11. Identify developing emergency situations, initiate appropriate action, and assist in treatment of the patient.

12. Discuss methods and types of documentation used in the OR.

E 13. Discuss the relationship between patient safety and the surgical environment.

■ Select Key Terms

Define the following:

1. apical pulse _____

   _____

2. autologous _____

   _____

3. cardiac dysrhythmia _____

   _____

4. catheterization _____

   _____

5. CPR _____

   _____

6. dyspnea _____

   _____

7. hemolysis _____

   _____

8. hemostasis _____

   _____

9. hemostat _____

   _____

10. homologous _____

    _____

11. informed consent _____

    _____

12. laser _____

    _____

13. NPO _____

    _____

14. prep _____

    _____

15. prone _____

    _____

16. pulse oximeter _____

    _____

17. Rh factor _____

    _____

18. sedation _____

    _____

19. shock _____

    _____

20. suction _____

    _____

21. supine _____

    _____

22. tourniquet _____

    _____

23. vital signs _____

    _____

■ **Case Studies**

☐ **CASE STUDY 1**

Viorel is a 10-year-old male who has been adopted. He is scheduled for a right inguinal herniorrhaphy.

1. Who has the authority to sign Viorel's operative consent?

_____

_____

_____

_____

2. In what position will Viorel be placed for the herniorrhaphy?

_____

_____

_____

_____

3. Describe the anatomical area that will be prepped.

_____

_____

_____

_____

4. Are any special considerations necesssary to accommodate Viorel's age?

_____

_____

_____

_____

☐

☐ CASE STUDY 2

After Virginia-May was placed on the operating table, it was discovered that her surgeon would be delayed by approximately 15 minutes. Virginia-May is 67 years old and is scheduled for a vaginal hysterectomy. She is very apprehensive.

1. What steps can be taken to help Virginia-May feel more comfortable?

   _____

   _____

   _____

   _____

2. Should the operating team continue with the preparations? For example, should she be anesthetized and positioned?

   _____

   _____

   _____

   _____

   ☐

Vital Signs – Temperature

Student Name _____ Date _____

Instructor _____

Procedural Step	Adequate	Needs Review
1. Student is able to state purpose for temperature monitoring		
2. Wash hands (Standard Precautions)		
3. Equipment and supplies are assembled		
4. Equipment prepared		
5. Identify patient, self, and explain procedure (if applicable)		
6. Position patient (if necessary)		
7. Place temperature probe		
8. Probe remains in position for prescribed amount of time		
9. Hold temperature probe in place (if necessary)		
10. Carefully remove temperature probe		
11. Read thermometer		
12. Wash hands (Standard Precautions)		
13. Record or report findings		
14. Care for equipment as needed		

Comments _____

_____

_____

_____

Vital Signs – Pulse

Student Name _____ Date _____

Instructor _____

Procedural Step	Adequate	Needs Review
1. Student is able to state purpose for pulse measurement		
2. Wash hands (Standard Precautions)		
3. Equipment and supplies are assembled		
4. Identify patient, self, and explain procedure (if applicable)		
5. Position patient (if necessary)		
6. Locate site		
7. Compress artery (or listen with stethoscope)		
8. Note time		
9. Count pulse rate and note rhythm, volume, and condition of the arterial wall		
10. Wash hands (Standard Precautions)		
11. Record or report findings		
12. Care for equipment as needed		

Comments _____

_____

_____

_____

Skill Assessment 8-3

Vital Signs – Respiration

Student Name _____   Date _____

Instructor _____

Procedural Step	Adequate	Needs Review
1. Student is able to state purpose of respiration monitoring		
2. Student is able to state normal respiration values, identify an abnormality, and explain the implications of an abnormality		
3. Wash hands (Standard Precautions)		
4. Equipment and supplies are assembled		
5. Identify patient, self, and explain procedure (if applicable)		
6. Position patient (if necessary)		
7. Obtain respiratory rate, depth, rhythm, and breath sounds		
8. Wash hands (Standard Precautions, if necessary)		
9. Record or report findings		
10. Care for equipment as needed		

Comments _____

_____

_____

_____

Vital Signs – Blood Pressure

Student Name _____ Date _____

Instructor _____

Procedural Step	Adequate	Needs Review
1. Student is able to state purpose for blood pressure monitoring		
2. Student is able to state normal blood pressure values, identify an abnormality, and explain the implications of an abnormality		
3. Wash hands (Standard Precautions)		
4. Equipment and supplies are assembled		
5. Identify patient, self, and explain procedure (if applicable)		
6. Position patient and expose site (if necessary)		
7. Apply blood pressure cuff		
8. Place stethoscope		
9. Inflate blood pressure cuff		
10. Deflate blood pressure cuff slowly, while listening for Korotkoff's sounds		
11. Continue deflation of blood pressure cuff. Continue to note sounds		
12. Complete deflation of cuff and remove cuff (if situation allows)		
13. Wash hands (Standard Precautions)		
14. Record or report findings		
15. Care for equipment as needed		

Comments _____

_____

_____

_____

Glove Oneself – Open Glove Technique
(Not Recommended When Wearing a Sterile Gown)

Student Name _____ Date _____

Instructor _____

Procedural Step	Adequate	Needs Review
1. Student is able to state purpose for application of sterile gloves		
2. Student is able to give several examples of situations in which the open glove technique will be necessary		
3. Wash hands (Standard Precautions)		
4. Equipment and supplies are assembled		
5. Remove outer wrapper		
6. Open inner wrapper		
7. Secure first glove from wrapper		
8. Apply first glove		
9. Secure second glove from wrapper		
10. Apply second glove		
11. Keep gloved hands sterile		

Comments _____

_____

_____

_____

Remove Soiled Gloves

Student Name _____ Date _____

Instructor _____

Procedural Step	Adequate	Needs Review
1. Student is able to state purpose for using correct glove removal technique		
2. Student is able to give examples of several situations in which this technique will be employed		
3. Equipment and supplies are assembled		
4. Grasp palm of glove to be removed first with opposite hand		
5. Remove first glove		
6. Keep removed glove in hand that remains gloved		
7. Begin to remove second glove		
8. Contain first glove inside of inverted second glove		
9. Finish removal of second glove		
10. Properly dispose of gloves		
11. Wash hands (Standard Precautions)		

Comments _____

_____

_____

_____

Urinary Catheterization
(Male or Female)

Student Name _____ Date _____

Instructor _____

Procedural Step	Adequate	Needs Review
1. Student is able to define urinary catheterization		
2. Student is able to state purpose for urinary catheterization		
3. Student is able to identify several situations in which urinary catheterization will be needed		
4. Student is able to identify different types of equipment that may be needed and state examples of when each may be used		
5. Wash hands (Standard Precautions)		
6. Equipment and supplies are assembled		
7. Identify patient, self, and explain procedure (if applicable)		
8. Position and expose patient		
9. Provide adequate lighting		
10. Remove protective cover and open catheter kit		
11. Don sterile gloves		
12. Organize supplies within sterile field		
13. Apply sterile drapes		
14. Cleanse meatus		
15. Insert catheter		
16. Inflate balloon		
17. Position catheter		
18. Care for patient and supplies as needed		
19. Wash hands (Standard Precautions)		
20. Document procedure		

Comments _____

_____

_____

Skin Prep

Student Name _____   Date _____

Instructor _____

Procedural Step	Adequate	Needs Review
1. Student is able to define surgical skin prep		
2. Student is able to state purpose for surgical skin prep		
3. Student is able to identify several situations that will require skin prep		
4. Student is able to identify different types of equipment and supplies that may be needed		
5. Wash hands (Standard Precautions)		
6. Equipment and supplies are assembled		
7. Identify patient, self, and explain procedure (if applicable)		
8. Position and expose patient		
9. Provide adequate lighting		
10. Open prep set		
11. Don sterile gloves		
12. Organize supplies within sterile field		
13. Apply sterile drapes		
14. Apply antiseptic solution to patient's skin		
15. Dry		
16. Apply "paint"		
17. Care for patient and supplies as needed		
18. Wash hands (Standard Precautions)		
19. Document procedure		

Comments _____

_____

_____

_____

CHAPTER 9

Surgical Pharmacology and Anesthesia

OBJECTIVES

After studying this chapter, the reader should be able to:

C 1. Define general terminology and abbreviations associated with pharmacology and anesthesia.

2. Describe the action, uses, and modes of administration of drugs and anesthetic agents used in the care of the surgical patient.

3. Describe the side effects and contraindications for use of drugs and anesthetic agents.

4. Describe the factors that influence anesthesia selection for individual patients.

A 5. Demonstrate safe practice in transferring drugs and solutions from the nonsterile area to the sterile field.

6. Demonstrate the procedure for identifying a drug or solution on the sterile field.

7. Explain how sterile technique is used in relation to certain anesthesia procedures.

R 8. Convert equivalents from one system to another and accurately identify, mix, and measure drugs for patient use.

9. Explain the roles of the STSR and circulator during the administration of anesthesia.

E 10. Discuss care and precautions in identifying drugs and solutions in the OR.

11. List the equipment used as an adjunct to anesthesia.

■ Select Key Terms

Define the following:

1. agonist _____

_____

2. amnesia _____

_____

3. anaphylaxis _____

_____

4. anesthesia _____

_____

5. antagonist _____

_____

6. antimuscarinic _____

_____

7. aspiration _____

_____

8. biotechnology _____

_____

9. buccal _____

_____

10. capnography _____

_____

11. contraindication _____

_____

12. doppler _____

_____

13. drug _____

_____

14. generic _____

_____

15. homeostasis _____

_____

16. hypnosis _____

_____

17. iatrogenic _____

_____

18. indication _____

_____

19. induction _____

_____

20. intra-articular _____

_____

21. laryngospasm _____

_____

22. NPO _____

_____

23. PACU _____

_____

24. parenteral _____

_____

25. pharmacodynamics _____

_____

26. pharmacokinetics _____

_____

27. pharmacology _____

_____

28. prophylaxis _____

_____

29. topical _____

_____

30. volatile agents _____

_____

■ Exercise A – Start and Maintain a Medication File

The student will keep an ongoing file of medications commonly used showing: Name of Drug—Generic Name (Trade Name), Drug Classification, Kinetics (drug action), Route(s) of Administration, Possible Iatrogenic, Adverse, or Idiosyncratic Reactions and Contraindications. (Index cards work well for this exercise.)

Additionally, the instructor may have the student include on the back of the card: Usual Dosages, Special Administration and Storage Instructions, Antagonist, Drug Interactions, Overdose Symptoms and Management, Preoperative Instructions, Pain Management, and Typical Onset, Peak Effect, and Duration Times.

Sample:

front

Drug Name: **Drug Classification:**

Drug Action: **Route(s) of Administration:**

Possible Iatrogenic, Adverse, or Idiosyncratic Reactions:

Contraindications:

back

Antagonist: **Special Administration and Storage Instructions:**

Usual Dosages: **Onset:**

Peak Effect:

Preoperatively: **Duration Time:**

Pain Management:

Drug Interactions:
MAO Inhibitors:
Overdose Symptoms:
Overdose Management:

■ Exercise B – Metric Conversions

Perform the following computations and exercises. Refer to Table 9-3 in the textbook if necessary.

1. Identify the following abbreviations.

   A. C   _____

   B. m   _____

   C. kg   _____

   D. L   _____

   E. μL   _____

   F. F   _____

   G. mm   _____

   H. mg   _____

   I. g   _____

   J. dL   _____

   K. m   _____

   L. μg   _____

   M. mL   _____

   N. cm   _____

   O. km   _____

   P. cc   _____

2. Calculate the following weight conversions.

   A. 14 lb =   _____ kg

   B. 123 lb =   _____ kg

   C. 46 kg =   _____ lb

   D. 78 kg =   _____ lb

   E. 4000 g =   _____ kg

   F. 4000 g =   _____ lb

   G. 1 g =   _____ mg

   H. 2000 mg = _____ oz

   I. 4 oz =   _____ g

   J. 114 g =   _____ mg

3. Calculate the following length conversions.

   A. 1 km =   _____ m

   B. 1000 m =   _____ miles

   C. 4 miles = _____ km

   D. 2 m =   _____ inches

   E. 17 inches = _____ cm

   F. 30 mm =   _____ inches

   G. 100 cm =   _____ inches

   H. 1 inch =   _____ cm

   I. 1 inch =   _____ mm

   J. 1 yard =   _____ cm

4. Calculate the following volume conversions.

   A. 1 mL =   _____ cc

   B. 4 cc =   _____ mL

   C. 2 oz =   _____ cc

   D. 5 liters = _____ cc

   E. 1 dL =   _____ mL

   F. 0.102 oz = _____ mL

   G. 500 cc =   _____ L

   H. 0.75 L =   _____ cc

   I. 0.034 oz = _____ cc

   J. 12 mL =   _____ oz

5. Calculate the following temperature conversions.

   A. 4°C =   _____ F

   B. 32°F =   _____ C

   C. 98.6°F =   _____ C

   D. 0°F =   _____ C

   E. 18°C =   _____ F

   F. 101°F =   _____ C

   G. 104°F =   _____ C

   H. 212°F =   _____ C

   I. 81°C =   _____ F

   J. 91.4°F =   _____ C

■ Exercise C – Identification

1. The trade names for several commonly used medications are listed. Provide the generic name.

   A. Ancef _____

   B. Anectine _____

   C. Coumadin _____

   D. Dantrium _____

   E. Decadron _____

   F. Demerol _____

   G. Forane _____

   H. Gelfoam _____

   I. Humulin _____

   J. Kantrex _____

   K. Lasix _____

   L. Marcaine _____

   M. Miochol _____

   N. Narcan _____

   O. Pitocin _____

   P. Robinul _____

   Q. Sublimaze _____

   R. Tagamet _____

   S. Toradol _____

   T. Tracrium _____

   U. Tylenol _____

   V. Valium _____

   W. Versed _____

   X. Wydase _____

2. Identify the components of the syringe shown in Figure 9-1.

   A. _____ D. _____

   B. _____ E. _____

   C. _____

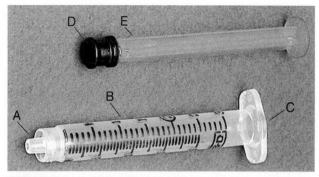

Figure 9-1

3. Identify the components of the needle shown in Figure 9-2.

   A. _____ D. _____

   B. _____ E. _____

   C. _____ F _____

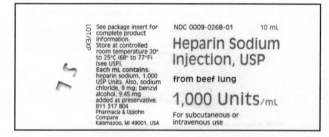

Figure 9-2

4. The physician has ordered 5,000 units of heparin. What volume of heparin will be needed? Use the medication labels pictured in Figure 9-3 to determine your answer. _____

   _____

   _____

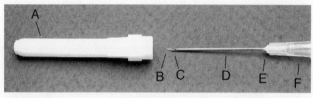

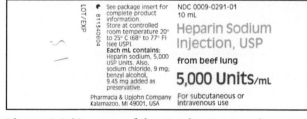

Figure 9-3 (Courtesy of the Upjohn Company)

5. From which source is heparin derived? _____

_____

6. The surgeon preference card calls for topical thrombin. Where will the STSR initially locate the medication? _____

_____

7. In which drug form is topical thrombin manufactured? _____

_____

8. What must be done to prepare the medication for use? _____

_____

9. What unit of measure is used to determine the dosage of topical thrombin? Use the medication label pictured in Figure 9-4 to determine your answer. _____

_____

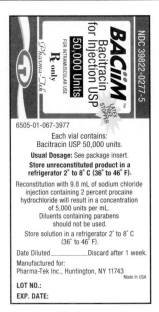

Figure 9-5 (Courtesy of Pharma-Tek, Inc.)

14. Cocaine HCl 4% has been ordered as a local anesthetic for a patient having nasal surgery. Will the cocaine be injected? _____

_____

15. What is the drug classification for cocaine? _____

_____

16. If any cocaine remains at the end of the procedure, is any special procedure necessary to ensure proper disposal? Why? _____

_____

17. The physician preference card calls for 1 g of kanamycin. How many vials of kanamycin will be needed? Use the medication label in Figure 9-6 to determine your answer. _____

_____

18. What is the drug classification for kanamycin?

_____

Figure 9-4 (Courtesy of Jones Pharma)

10. The physician has ordered 100,000 units of bacitracin, diluted in 1,000 cc of saline, for irrigation of the abdominal cavity. How many vials of bacitracin will be needed? Use the medication label pictured in Figure 9-5 to determine your answer. _____

_____

11. In which drug form is bacitracin manufactured?

_____

12. What must be done to prepare bacitracin for use? _____

_____

13. How will the bacitracin/saline solution be introduced into the abdominal cavity? What supplies will be necessary? _____

_____

Figure 9-6 (Courtesy of Apothecon)

19. For what purpose would kanamycin be ordered?

   _____

20. What is the drug classification for oxytocin?

   _____

21. In what situation(s) in the operating room is the use of oxytocin indicated? _____

   _____

22. The surgeon has requested that the STSR have 20 units of oxytocin available on the sterile field. How many vials will be necessary? Use the medication label in Figure 9-7 to determine your answer. _____

   _____

23. Via which route(s) is oxytocin administered?

   _____

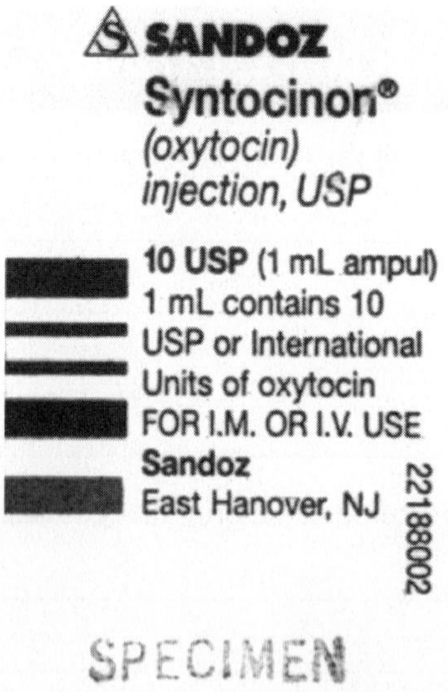

△ SANDOZ

Syntocinon®
(oxytocin)
injection, USP

10 USP (1 mL ampul)
1 mL contains 10
USP or International
Units of oxytocin
FOR I.M. OR I.V. USE
Sandoz
East Hanover, NJ   22188002

SPECIMEN

Figure 9-7 (Courtesy of Novartis Pharmaceuticals Corp.)

■ Case Studies

□ CASE STUDY 1

Amanda, a 22-month-old female, is scheduled to have a percutaneous liver biopsy under general anesthesia at 7:30 AM. Her mother states that she has been NPO since last evening when she drank a bottle of 2% milk about 8:00 PM.

1. Why will Amanda be having a general anesthetic?

   _____

   _____

   _____

   _____

2. Has Amanda been NPO for an adequate amount of time?

   _____

   _____

   _____

   _____

(continues)

☐ **CASE STUDY 1** (*continued*)

3. How will the anesthetist determine the approximate size of Amanda's trachea?

_____

_____

_____

_____

4. How are pediatric drug dosages calculated?

_____

_____

_____

_____

5. What special anesthesia equipment, if any, will be needed to care for Amanda?

_____

_____

_____

_____

_____

☐

☐ **CASE STUDY 2**

Tony, an 86-year-old male, is scheduled for a ventral herniorrhaphy with general anesthesia. An IV line has been inserted in Tony's left forearm. You have been asked to assist the anesthesiologist and the circulator as they position Tony on the operating table and apply the devices that will be used to monitor his condition while he is anesthetized.

1. Will Tony's position remain the same for his anesthetic administration and the procedure? What position(s) will be necessary?

_____

_____

_____

_____

☐ CASE STUDY 2 (*continued*)

2. Place the following monitors and safety devices on Tony. Indicate placement by writing the corresponding letters on the diagram of Tony (Figure 9-8). Provide your rationale for each placement decision.

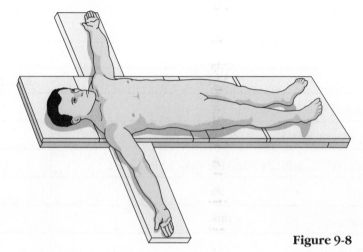

Figure 9-8

A. IV— _____

_____

B. Thermometer— _____

_____

C. Blood Pressure Cuff— _____

_____

D. Pulse Oximeter— _____

_____

E. Safety Strap— _____

_____

F. Electrosurgical Grounding Pad— _____

_____

G. 5-Lead ECG Electrodes— _____

_____

3. Show the area that will be prepped by lightly shading it in on Tony's figure. Why is it important to consider the skin prep when placing monitors?

_____

_____

_____

☐

Sellick's Maneuver

Student Name _____ Date _____

Instructor _____

Procedural Step	Adequate	Needs Review
1. Student is able to define Sellick's Maneuver		
2. Verbalize purpose of Sellick's Maneuver		
3. Give two examples in which Sellick's Maneuver may be indicated		
4. Position self properly		
5. Identify relevant anatomy		
6. Position hand properly		
7. Apply adequate pressure		
8. Maintain cricoid pressure until asked to release		

Comments _____

_____

_____

_____

Draw Up Medication in a Syringe (Off the Sterile Field)

Student Name _____ Date _____

Instructor _____

Procedural Step	Adequate	Needs Review
1. Student is able to provide pertinent information about the medication ordered		
2. Secure the ordered medication and all necessary supplies		
3. Verify that the "five rights" are met		
4. Verify that patient is not allergic to ordered medication		
5. Prepare medication container for withdrawal of medication		
6. Withdraw medication from container		
7. Needle for injection is applied to the syringe		
8. Medication label information is rechecked for accuracy		
9. Medication is labeled according to facility policy		

Comments _____

_____

_____

_____

Draw Up Medication in a Syringe (Into the Sterile Field)

Student Name _____ Date _____

Instructor _____

Procedural Step	Adequate	Needs Review
1. Student is able to provide pertinent information about the medication ordered		
2. Secure the ordered medication and all necessary supplies		
3. Verify that the "five rights" are met		
4. Verify that patient is not allergic to ordered medication		
5. Circulator prepares medication container for withdrawal of medication		
6. STSR and circulator visually and verbally identify medication		
7. STSR withdraws medication from container		
8. STSR and circulator visually and verbally identify medication		
9. Needle for injection is applied to the syringe (if necessary)		
10. Medication is labeled according to facility policy		
11. Medication is passed to surgeon when requested and properly verbally identified		

Comments _____

_____

_____

_____

Accept Medication Into the Sterile Field (Into a Container)

Student Name _____ Date _____

Instructor _____

Procedural Step	Adequate	Needs Review
1. Student is able to provide pertinent information about the medication ordered		
2. Secure the ordered medication and all necessary supplies		
3. Verify that the "five rights" are met		
4. Verify that patient is not allergic to ordered medication		
5. Circulator prepares medication for transfer to the sterile field		
6. STSR and circulator visually and verbally identify medication		
7. STSR presents container for acceptance of medication		
8. Medication is transferred to sterile field		
9. STSR and circulator visually and verbally identify medication		
10. Medication is correctly diluted (if necessary)		
11. Medication container is labeled according to facility policy		
12. Medication is prepared for use and additionally labeled (if necessary)		
13. Medication is passed to surgeon when requested and properly verbally identified		

Comments _____

_____

_____

_____

CHAPTER 10

Instrumentation, Equipment, and Supplies

OBJECTIVES

After studying this chapter, the reader should be able to:

C 1. Discuss the relationship between instrumentation, equipment, and supplies and quality patient care in the OR.

A 2. Identify items that require sterilization prior to use in the sterile field.

R 3. Identify basic instruments by type, function, and name.

4. Demonstrate proper care, handling, and assembly of instruments.

5. Identify types of special equipment utilized in OR practice and demonstrate proper care, handling techniques, and safety precautions.

6. Identify the names and functions of accessory equipment and demonstrate proper care, handling, and assembly.

7. Identify and prepare supplies used in the OR.

E 8. Discuss the relationship between instruments, equipment, and supplies and the OR environment as related to safety.

■ Select Key Words
Define the following:

1. ancillary _____

_____

2. aperture _____

_____

3. bipolar electrosurgery _____

_____

4. capillary action_____

_____

5. catheter_____

_____

6. cottonoid _____

_____

7. cryo- _____

_____

8. defibrillator_____

_____

9. drain _____

_____

10. fenestration_____

_____

11. insufflation _____

_____

12. irrigation _____

_____

13. magnification _____

_____

14. monopolar cautery _____

_____

15. Nd:YAG_____

_____

16. pneumatic_____

_____

17. resistance _____

_____

18. retract _____

_____

19. scalpel_____

_____

20. serrations _____

_____

21. stainless steel _____

_____

22. teeth _____

_____

23. tube_____

_____

24. ureteral _____

_____

25. urethral_____

_____

■ **Exercise A – Identification**

1. Identify the components of the instrument shown in Figure 10-1.

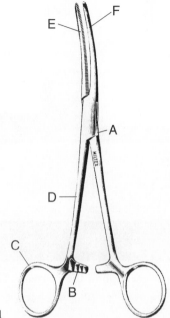

Figure 10-1

A. _____

B. _____

C. _____

D. _____

E. _____

F. _____

2. Classify the instruments listed using the following designations:

Accessory   Clamping/Occluding   Cutting   Dilating
Grasping/Holding   Probing   Retracting
Suctioning   Suturing

A. #3 Knife Handle   _____

B. Allis   _____

C. Babcock   _____

D. Crile

E. Deaver   _____

F. Debakey Tissue Forceps   _____

G. Kocher   _____

H. Metzenbaum   _____

I. Mosquito   _____

J. Needle Holder   _____

K. Poole   _____

L. Richardson   _____

M. Towel Clamp   _____

N. Yankauer   _____

3. Organize the following instruments by size from shortest/smallest to longest/largest.

A. _____   Crile

B. _____   Mosquito

C. _____   Pean

D. _____   Schnidt

4. A #20 knife blade fits on a # _____ knife handle.

5. A #15 knife blade fits on a # _____ knife handle.

6. An oscillating saw uses a(n) _____ motion.

7. A reciprocating saw uses a(n) _____ motion.

8. The acronym "laser" represents _____

9. Trace the path of the electrical current when a unipolar electrosurgical unit is in use by placing the following elements in the correct order.

A. _____   Active Electrode

B. _____   Dispersive Electrode

C. _____   Generator

D. _____   Generator

E. _____   Ground

F. _____   Patient

10. Identify the types of sponges shown in Figure 10-2.

    A. _____

    B. _____

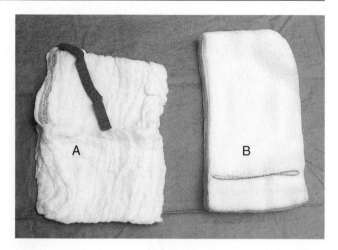

Figure 10-2

■ Case Studies

Edward has been assigned to prepare the Cysto Room for a transurethral resection of the prostate (TURP) using the Nd:YAG laser.

1. What does Nd:YAG represent? _____

   _____

   _____

   _____

   _____

2. What precautions must be taken to protect the patient and staff from the laser beam? _____

   _____

   _____

   _____

   _____

3. Will the laser be attached to the endoscope?

   _____

   _____

   _____

   _____

                                                                              ☐

☐ CASE STUDY 2

Madelena is preparing the OR for a neurosurgical procedure (carpal tunnel release). Both the unipolar and bipolar electrosurgical units are requested on the surgeon's preference card.

1. Will Madelena need two grounding pads (dispersive electrodes)? Why or why not? _____

_____

_____

_____

_____

2. The patient will be placed in the supine position for the procedure. What anatomic site is the most likely place to affix the grounding pad(s)?_____

_____

_____

_____

3. The surgeon's preference card requests that a tourniquet be available for the procedure. List at least three items that Madelena will need to facilitate the use of the tourniquet. _____

_____

_____

_____

_____

☐

Assemble an Instrument Set

Student Name _____ Date _____

Instructor _____

Procedural Step	Adequate	Needs Review
1. Student is able to state purpose for assembling an instrument set in prescribed manner		
2. Appropriate attire		
3. Wash hands (Standard Precautions)		
4. Equipment and supplies assembled		
5. Organize workspace		
6. Assemble set		
7. Sign/initial count sheet/instrument list		
8. Place internal indicator		
9. Proceed with other tasks		

Comments _____

_____

_____

_____

Instrument Handling – Load, Pass, and Unload a Scalpel Handle

Student Name _____ Date _____

Instructor _____

Procedural Step	Adequate	Needs Review
1. Equipment and supplies assembled		
2. Student selects necessary items		
3. Scalpel blade is secured		
4. Blade is applied to handle		
5. Proceed with case preparation or case		
6. Scalpel is held in safe manner		
7. Scalpel is passed or placed for transfer		
8. Scalpel is retrieved		
9. Blade is removed from handle		
10. Discard blade		
11. Proceed with case or case breakdown		

Comments _____

_____

_____

_____

Instrument Handling – Recognize, Prepare, and Pass Various Types of Instruments (Sharps, Scissors, Tissue Forceps, Ringed Instruments, and Retractors)

Student Name _____ Date _____

Instructor _____

Procedural Step	Adequate	Needs Review
1. Equipment and supplies assembled		
2. Mayo stand is set up		
3. Student is able to recognize instruments by name		
4. Student secures instrument requested		
5. Pass sharp instruments or supplies		
6. Pass scissors		
7. Pass tissue forceps		
8. Pass ringed instrument(s)		
9. Pass retractor(s)		
10. Return items to storage location		
11. Attend to other intraoperative actions as needed		

Comments _____

_____

_____

_____

CHAPTER 11

Wound Healing, Sutures, Needles, and Stapling Devices

OBJECTIVES

After studying this chapter, the reader should be able to:

C
1. Define terms relevant to wound healing.
2. List the possible complications of wound healing.

A
3. Explain the classifications of surgical wounds.
4. Define and give examples of types of traumatic wounds.
5. List the factors that influence healing and describe the manner in which they affect the healing process.

R
6. Describe the characteristics of inflammation.
7. List and define common suture terms.
8. Identify suture materials and stapling devices and their usage.
9. Describe the types, characteristics, and uses of natural and synthetic absorbable suture materials.
10. List and describe the common natural and synthetic nonabsorbable sutures, stating their sources, common trade names, and uses.
11. Discuss preparation and handling techniques for suturing and stapling devices, and list the factors relating to the choice of each.
12. List and define common suture techniques.
13. Discuss the basic uses and advantages of stapling instruments.
14. Identify, describe the use of, and demonstrate proper handling of the various types of surgical needles.

E
15. List the types of injury that cause damage to tissues.
16. List the characteristics of the types of healing.
17. Describe the stages/phases of wound healing.

Select Key Terms

Define the following:

1. adhesion _____

_____

2. anastomosis _____

_____

3. approximated _____

_____

4. chromic gut _____

_____

5. chronic wound _____

_____

6. cicatrix _____

_____

7. dead space _____

_____

8. debridement _____

_____

9. dehiscence _____

_____

10. devitalized _____

_____

11. evisceration _____

_____

12. first intention _____

_____

13. fray _____

_____

14. French-eyed needle _____

_____

15. friable _____

16. herniation _____

_____

17. immunosuppressed patient _____

_____

18. inflammation _____

_____

19. laceration _____

_____

20. ligate _____

_____

21. monofilament _____

_____

22. packing _____

_____

23. primary suture line _____

_____

24. PTFE _____

_____

25. second intention _____

_____

26. secondary suture line _____

_____

27. swaged _____

_____

28. tensile strength _____

_____

29. third intention _____

_____

30. vessel loop _____

_____

■ Case Studies

□ CASE STUDY 1

James, a 12-year-old male, lost control of his trail bike while riding on a course that he and some friends constructed in a vacant lot. He flew over the handle-bars into the dirt onto his left arm. His arm is broken, and the bone is sticking out through the skin. It is 10:00 AM.

1. James has suffered a traumatic injury to his left arm. What classification(s) does his wound fall into?_____

   _____

   _____

   _____

   _____

2. James was immediately taken to the Urgent Care Center. It is determined that James will need surgical treatment and will be transferred by ambulance to the nearest hospital, which is 150 miles away. The surgery is scheduled for 4:00 PM. How will the surgical wound be classified? Why?_____

   _____

   _____

   _____

   _____

3. Is James at risk for surgical site infection? Why? What steps can be taken to minimize the risk of SSI? _____

   _____

   _____

   _____

   _____

☐ **CASE STUDY 2**

Dorothea just had her ruptured appendix removed. The skin and subcutaneous layers of her wound have been left open. Her surgeon told her that if her wound showed no signs of infection in 5 days he would finish the closure.

1. Why did the surgeon leave the wound partially open? In its present condition, by what method is the wound expected to heal? _____

    _____

    _____

    _____

    _____

2. What signs will the surgeon use to determine if Dorothea's wound may be closed in 5 days?_____

    _____

    _____

    _____

    _____

3. If the wound can be closed in 5 days, what type of healing will then be expected? Is the tissue expected to regain normal tensile strength?_____

    _____

    _____

    _____

    _____

☐

Suture/Needle/Staple Handling – Load, Pass, and Unload a Needle Holder

Student Name _____ Date _____

Instructor _____

Procedural Step	Adequate	Needs Review
1. Equipment and supplies assembled		
2. Select necessary items		
3. Open suture packet		
4. Needle holder is applied		
5. Suture is removed from packet		
6. Pass suture		
7. Companion instruments passed		
8. Suture is retrieved		
9. Needle holder is unloaded		
10. Return items to storage location		
11. Attend to other intraoperative actions as needed		

Comments _____

_____

_____

_____

Suture/Needle/Staple Handling – Load Empty Needle, Thread Suture, Pass, and Reload

Student Name _____ Date _____

Instructor _____

Procedural Step	Adequate	Needs Review
1. Equipment and supplies assembled		
2. Select necessary items		
3. Open suture packet		
4. Needle is placed in needle holder		
5. Needle holder is moved to left hand		
6. Suture is threaded		
7. Pass suture		
8. Companion instruments passed		
9. Needle is retrieved		
10. Reset needle and reload (if necessary)		
11. Needle holder is unloaded		
12. Return items to storage location		
13. Attend to other intraoperative actions as needed		

Comments _____

_____

_____

_____

Suture/Needle/Staple Handling – Pass Ties
(Includes Reel, Free Ties, and Ties on a Pass)

Student Name _____ Date _____

Instructor _____

Procedural Step	Adequate	Needs Review
1. Equipment and supplies assembled		
2. Select necessary items		
3. Prepare, pass, and retrieve reel		
4. Prepare and pass free tie		
5. Prepare and pass tie on a pass		
6. Attend to other intraoperative actions as needed		

Comments _____

_____

_____

_____

Suture/Needle/Staple Handling – Load, Pass, and Unload Various Types of Stapling/Clipping Devices

Student Name _____ Date _____

Instructor _____

Procedural Step	Adequate	Needs Review
1. Equipment and supplies assembled		
2. Select necessary items		
3. Item is prepared for use		
4. Item is passed		
5. Item is retrieved		
6. Attend to other intraoperative actions as needed		

Comments _____

_____

_____

_____

CHAPTER 12

Surgical Case Management

OBJECTIVES

After studying this chapter, the reader should be able to:

C 1. Describe the role of the STSR in caring for the surgical patient.

A 2. Demonstrate techniques of opening and preparing supplies and instruments needed for any operative procedure with the maintenance of sterile technique at all times.

3. Demonstrate the proper techniques for the surgical hand scrub, gowning, gloving, and assisting team members.

4. Demonstrate the proper technique for preparing supplies and instruments on a sterile field.

R 5. Demonstrate and explain in detail the procedure for counting instruments, sponges, needles, and other items on the sterile field.

6. Demonstrate the initial steps for starting a procedure.

7. Demonstrate intraoperative handling of sterile equipment and supplies.

E 8. Explain and demonstrate postoperative routines.

■ Select Key Terms

Define the following:

1. adhesive _____

_____

2. anticipate _____

_____

3. antimicrobial _____

_____

4. biohazard _____

_____

5. circumferentially _____

_____

6. count _____

_____

7. craniotomy _____

_____

8. cylindrical _____

_____

9. donning _____

_____

10. foreign body _____

_____

11. handwash _____

_____

12. indicator _____

_____

13. lap sponge _____

_____

14. mask _____

_____

15. neutral zone _____

_____

16. pathology _____

_____

17. PPE _____

_____

18. resident organisms _____

_____

19. scrub (sterile) attire _____

_____

20. sterile team member _____

_____

21. stockinette _____

_____

22. surgeon's preference card _____

_____

23. surgical scrub _____

_____

24. transient organisms _____

_____

25. wraparound-style gown _____

_____

■ Case Studies

□ CASE STUDY 1

Sean is a student STSR for an LAVH. As he reaches for a supply item being handed by the circulator, his left glove touches the outside of the packet.

1. Does Sean have a problem? What is it?

     _____

     _____

     _____

     _____

2. What steps need to be taken to correct the problem?

     _____

     _____

     _____

     _____

3. Describe the procedure(s) for changing a contaminated glove.

     _____

     _____

     _____

     _____

□

☐ CASE STUDY 2

It is LuAnn's big day. She is scrubbing her first case as a student. She wants desperately to do everything right.

1. What type of surgical scrub should LuAnn perform? Why?

   _____

   _____

   _____

   _____

2. Describe the counted brush stroke method for a surgical scrub.

   _____

   _____

   _____

   _____

3. Which method of self-gloving will LuAnn use after she has donned her sterile gown? Why?

   _____

   _____

   _____

   _____

   ☐

OR Attire

Student Name _____ Date _____

Instructor _____

Procedural Step	Adequate	Needs Review
1. Student is able to state purpose for wearing OR attire		
2. Student is able to state situations when variations in OR attire may occur		
3. Student is able to state when OR attire is to be worn		
4. Scrub suit		
5. No jewelry		
6. No cosmetics		
7. Hair cover		
8. Identification		
9. Radiation monitoring device		
10. Shoes appropriate to OR		
11. Shoe covers		
12. Mask		
13. Eyewear		

Comments _____

_____

_____

_____

Open Sterile Supplies – Back Table Pack

Student Name _____ Date _____

Instructor _____

Procedural Step	Adequate	Needs Review
1. Appropriate attire		
2. Wash hands (Standard Precautions)		
3. Equipment and supplies assembled		
4. Check integrity of package		
5. Remove dust cover		
6. Check integrity of inner package		
7. Orient pack on back table		
8. Open first fold and remove accessory items, if present		
9. Open second fold		
10. Open third fold		
11. Reposition self to open fourth fold		
12. Open fourth fold		
13. Proceed with case preparation		

Comments _____

_____

_____

_____

Open Sterile Supplies – Small Wrapped Package
(Such as Initial Gown – On Clean Surface)

Student Name _____ Date _____

Instructor _____

Procedural Step	Adequate	Needs Review
1. Appropriate attire		
2. Wash hands (Standard Precautions)		
3. Equipment and supplies assembled		
4. Check integrity of package		
5. Orient package on appropriate surface		
6. Open first fold		
7. Open second fold		
8. Open third fold		
9. Open fourth fold		
10. Proceed with case preparation		

Comments _____

_____

_____

_____

Open Sterile Supplies – Small Wrapped Package
(Onto Sterile Field or Secured by STSR)

Student Name _____ Date _____

Instructor _____

Procedural Step	Adequate	Needs Review
1. Appropriate attire		
2. Wash hands (Standard Precautions)		
3. Equipment and supplies assembled		
4. Check integrity of package		
5. Orient package properly in hand		
6. Open first fold, secure flap		
7. Open second fold, secure flap		
8. Open third fold, secure flap		
9. Open fourth fold, secure flap		
10. Approach sterile field/STSR		
11. Transfer item to sterile field/STSR		
12. Discard wrapper		
13. Proceed with case preparation		

Comments _____

_____

_____

_____

Open Sterile Supplies – Peel Pack

Student Name _____ Date _____

Instructor _____

Procedural Step	Adequate	Needs Review
1. Appropriate attire		
2. Wash hands (Standard Precautions)		
3. Equipment and supplies assembled		
4. Check integrity of package		
5. Orient package properly in both hands		
6. Slowly pull sides of peel pack away from each other		
7. Continue opening package		
8. Approach sterile field/STSR		
9. Transfer item to sterile field/STSR		
10. Discard wrapper		
11. Proceed with case preparation		

Comments _____

_____

_____

_____

Open Sterile Supplies – Instrument Set (Container System)

Student Name _____ Date _____

Instructor _____

Procedural Step	Adequate	Needs Review
1. Appropriate attire		
2. Wash hands (Standard Precautions)		
3. Equipment and supplies assembled		
4. Check integrity of container		
5. Place instrument container on suitable surface		
6. Remove seals		
7. Release lid		
8. Lift lid		
9. Inspect interior of container		
10. Inspect lid		
11. Set lid in convenient location		
12. Proceed with case preparation		

Comments _____

_____

_____

_____

Open Sterile Supplies – Pour Sterile Solution

Student Name _____ Date _____

Instructor _____

Procedural Step	Adequate	Needs Review
1. Student is able to provide pertinent information about the sterile solution ordered		
2. Appropriate attire		
3. Wash hands (Standard Precautions)		
4. Equipment and supplies assembled		
5. Verify that the "five rights" are met		
6. Verify patient allergy status		
7. Remove protective outer seal from solution container		
8. Remove inner seal		
9. Approach sterile field		
10. STSR and circulator visually and verbally identify solution		
11. Pour sterile solution		
12. STSR and circulator visually and verbally identify solution		
13. Proceed with case preparation		

Comments _____

_____

_____

_____

Surgical Scrub – Counted Brush Stroke Method

Student Name _____ Date _____

Instructor _____

Procedural Step	Adequate	Needs Review
1. Student is able to define surgical scrub		
2. Student is able to state purpose for performing surgical scrub		
3. Appropriate attire		
4. Equipment and supplies are assembled		
5. Inspect integrity of hands and arms		
6. Open brush package		
7. Turn on water and adjust temperature		
8. Wet hands and arms, apply soap, lather		
9. Clean nails		
10. Rinse		
11. Secure and prepare brush		
12. Scrub nails of first hand		
13. Scrub fingers of first hand		
14. Scrub hand of first arm		
15. Scrub arm to 2″ above elbow of first arm		
16. Transfer brush to scrubbed hand and scrub opposite extremity		
17. Discard brush		
18. Rinse		
19. Proceed to OR		

Comments _____

_____

_____

_____

Skill Assessment 12-9

Gown – Self
(Dry, Don Gown and Gloves – Closed Glove Technique)

Student Name _____ Date _____

Instructor _____

Procedural Step	Adequate	Needs Review
1. Enter OR		
2. Secure towel		
3. Open towel		
4. Dry first hand and arm		
5. Transfer towel to opposite hand		
6. Dry opposite hand		
7. Discard towel		
8. Secure gown		
9. Unfold gown		
10. Don gown		
11. Secure first glove		
12. Position glove appropriately		
13. Don first glove		
14. Secure and don second glove		
15. Wrap around back of gown		
16. Remove lubricant (powder) from gloves		
17. Proceed with case preparation		

Comments _____

_____

_____

_____

Gown – Assist a Team Member
(Pass Towel, Apply Gown and Gloves – Open Glove Technique)

Student Name _____ Date _____

Instructor _____

Procedural Step	Adequate	Needs Review
1. Prepare items in advance of need		
2. Secure towel		
3. Open towel		
4. Present towel to team member		
5. Secure gown		
6. Unfold gown		
7. Present gown		
8. Secure right glove		
9. Prepare right glove		
10. Present right glove		
11. Secure, prepare, and present left glove		
12. Wrap around back of gown		
13. Remove lubricant (powder) from gloves		
14. Proceed with case preparation or case		

Comments _____

_____

_____

_____

Disrobe
(To Replace Sterile Attire During Case)

Student Name _____ Date _____

Instructor _____

Procedural Step	Adequate	Needs Review
1. Recognize that gloves and/or gown are contaminated during case		
2. Step away from sterile field and request new gown and appropriate size gloves		
3. Remain still, with back to circulator while gown is unfastened		
4. Face circulator; remain still while gown is removed		
5. Turn hands palm up and present one at a time to circulator (usually right hand first)		
6. Apply sterile gown and gloves		
7. Return to sterile field and continue with tasks		

Comments _____

_____

_____

_____

Disrobe
(End of Case)

Student Name _____ Date _____

Instructor _____

Procedural Step	Adequate	Needs Review
1. All tasks that require gown and gloves are complete		
2. Back of gown is unfastened		
3. Grasp gown near shoulders and roll away from self		
4. Remove gown (place gown in proper receptacle if feasible)		
5. Remove soiled gloves		
6. Grasp palm of glove to be removed first with opposite hand		
7. Remove first glove		
8. Keep removed glove in hand that remains gloved		
9. Begin to remove second glove		
10. Contain first glove inside of inverted second glove		
11. Finish removal of second glove		
12. Properly dispose of gown and gloves		
13. Wash hands (Standard Precautions)		

Comments _____

_____

_____

_____

Dress the Mayo Stand

Student Name _____ Date _____

Instructor _____

Procedural Step	Adequate	Needs Review
1. Equipment and supplies assembled		
2. Orient Mayo stand cover		
3. Insert hands in cuff of Mayo stand cover		
4. Secure folded edges of Mayo stand cover		
5. Approach Mayo stand		
6. Insert bare Mayo stand into prepared pocket of Mayo stand cover		
7. Slide Mayo stand cover onto Mayo stand		
8. Allow Mayo stand cover to unfold over back edge of stand		
9. Make final adjustments		
10. Place towels		
11. Proceed with case preparation		

Comments _____

_____

_____

_____

Skill Assessment 12-14

Fill a Bulb Syringe

Student Name _____ Date _____

Instructor _____

Procedural Step	Adequate	Needs Review
1. Equipment and supplies assembled		
2. Prepare bulb syringe		
3. Remove air		
4. Fill bulb syringe		
5. Proceed with case preparation or case		

Comments _____

_____

_____

_____

Remove Instrument Set from Container

Student Name _____ Date _____

Instructor _____

Procedural Step	Adequate	Needs Review
1. Equipment and supplies assembled		
2. Approach instrument container		
3. Secure instrument basket		
4. Step away from instrument container		
5. Place instrument basket on back table		
6. Proceed with case preparation or case		

Comments _____

_____

_____

_____

Case Management – Pre-Case Preparation
(Prior to Scrub)

Student Name _____ Date _____

Instructor _____

Procedural Step	Adequate	Needs Review
1. Appropriate attire		
2. Wash hands (Standard Precautions)		
3. Assignment received		
4. Secure surgeon preference card		
5. Locate case cart or assemble necessary items		
6. Verify that all items are present		
7. OR prepared for use		
8. Sterile items placed for use		
9. Open standard and specialty items		
10. Double-check supplies		
11. Proceed with case preparation		

Comments _____

_____

_____

_____

Case Management – Case Preparation
(Beginning with Surgical Scrub)

Student Name _____ Date _____

Instructor _____

Procedural Step	Adequate	Needs Review
1. Appropriate attire		
2. Sterility is maintained at all times		
3. Perform surgical scrub		
4. Proceed to OR		
5. Approach sterile field, secure towel, and dry self		
6. Don sterile gown		
7. Apply sterile gloves		
8. Prepare back table and basin set; dress Mayo stand		
9. Count necessary items		
10. Mayo stand prepared for use		
11. Preparation time less than 20 minutes		

Comments _____

_____

_____

_____

Case Management – Drape
(Basic Laparotomy)

Student Name _____ Date _____

Instructor _____

Procedural Step	Adequate	Needs Review
1. Equipment and supplies assembled		
2. Prepare drape materials		
3. Remain vigilant		
4. Report and correct problems immediately		
5. Hold drape materials at correct level		
6. Pass drape materials correctly		
7. Move safely between sterile fields		
8. Hand drapes in proper sequence		
9. Protect hands with drape cuff		
10. Communicate with team members as needed		
11. Other equipment is ready for placement		
12. Move furniture into position		
13. Proceed with case preparation or case		

Comments _____

_____

_____

_____

Case Management – Intraoperative Actions

Student Name _____ Date _____

Instructor _____

Procedural Step	Adequate	Needs Review
1. Equipment and supplies assembled		
2. Assist other team members to enter sterile field		
3. Perform tasks related to draping		
4. Place additional equipment on field as needed		
5. Move furniture into position		
6. Prepare field		
7. Pass scalpel		
8. Handle electrosurgical pencil properly		
9. Hand instruments correctly		
10. Prepare, identify, and handle all solutions correctly		
11. Prepare, identify, and handle all medications correctly		
12. Remove small sponges (if necessary)		
13. Respond to team member needs appropriately		
14. Communicate effectively with circulator		
15. Prepare, identify, and handle sutures and needles correctly		
16. Perform closing count(s)		
17. Report and correct problems immediately		
18. Maintain an orderly field		
19. Prepare for end of case		
20. Maintain sterile field until patient removed from OR		
21. Proceed with post-procedure actions		

Comments _____

_____

_____

Case Management – Post-Procedure Actions

Student Name _____ Date _____

Instructor _____

Procedural Step	Adequate	Needs Review
1. Maintain sterile field until patient removed from OR		
2. Remove drapes from patient		
3. Assist with patient care as needed		
4. Return to tasks related to breakdown of field		
5. Handle all materials safely		
6. Dispose of all sharps correctly		
7. Handle all biohazardous waste (linen and trash) correctly		
8. Follow policy for instrument care		
9. Remove gown and gloves properly		
10. Wash hands (Standard Precautions)		
11. Care for equipment as needed		
12. Follow OR cleaning/turn-over procedure		

Comments _____

_____

_____

_____

CHAPTER 13

Diagnostic Procedures

OBJECTIVES

After studying this chapter, the reader should be able to:

A 1. Apply knowledge of anatomy and physiology to determine which diagnostic examinations will be useful.

P 2. List the sources of patient data.

3. List and discuss techniques used to establish the diagnosis.

O 4. Determine which diagnostic procedures will require surgical intervention.

5. Identify the major indications for surgical intervention.

S 6. Understand the surgical technologist's role in caring for each specific type of specimen.

■ Select Key Terms

Define the following:

1. angina _____

_____

2. auscultation _____

_____

3. biopsy _____

_____

4. capnography _____

_____

5. C-arm _____

_____

6. cholangiography _____

_____

7. contrast media _____

_____

8. CSF _____

_____

9. cystoscopy _____

_____

10. ECG _____

_____

11. EEG _____

_____

12. frozen section _____

13. -gram _____

_____

14. Gram stain _____

_____

15. -graph _____

_____

16. indwelling _____

_____

17. isotope scanning _____

_____

18. obstruction _____

_____

19. palpation _____

_____

20. prosthesis _____

_____

21. Roentgenography _____

_____

22. sign _____

_____

23. symptom _____

_____

24. urinalysis (UA) _____

_____

25. ultrasonography _____

_____

■ **Exercise A – Anatomy**

1. Identify the structures of the biliary tract shown in Figure 13-1.

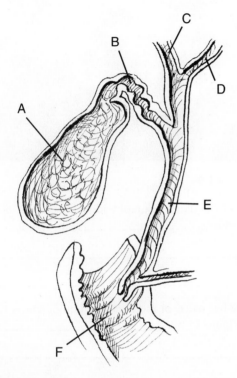

Figure 13-1

A. _____   B. _____

C. _____   D. _____

E. _____   F. _____

2. What type of radiographic exam would be used to visualize the structures of the biliary tract?

_____

_____

3. Identify the bony structures shown in Figure 13-2.

A. _____   B. _____

C. _____   D. _____

E. _____   F. _____

4. What radiographic view is shown in Figure 13-2, and which structure(s) is/are the primary focus of the exam? _____

_____

_____

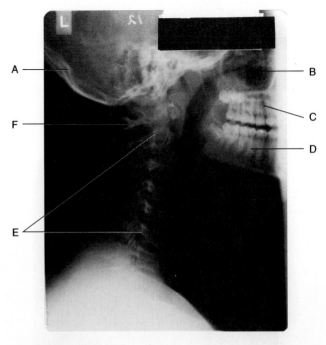

Figure 13-2

5. Identify the bony structures shown in Figure 13-3.

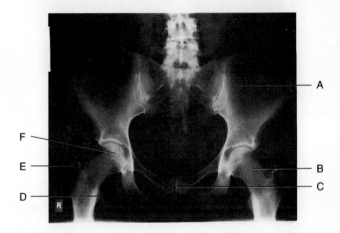

Figure 13-3

A. _____   B. _____

C. _____   D. _____

E. _____   F. _____

6. What radiographic view is shown in Figure 13-3?

_____

_____

7. In what position was the patient placed in order to obtain the radiographic view shown in Figure 13-3?

_____

_____

8. Identify the structures of the urinary system shown in Figure 13-4.

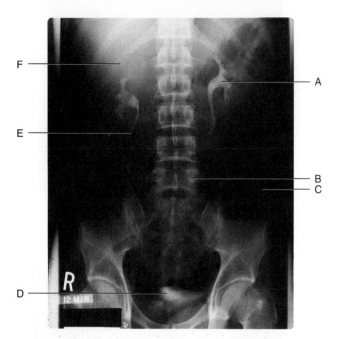

Figure 13-4

A. _____   B. _____

C. _____   D. _____

E. _____   F. _____

9. Has contrast been used to obtain the radiograph shown in Figure 13-4?_____

_____

_____

10. In what position was the patient placed in order to obtain the radiographic view shown in Figure 13-4?

_____

_____

11. Figure 13-5 shows an image of the liver. How was this image obtained? _____

_____

_____

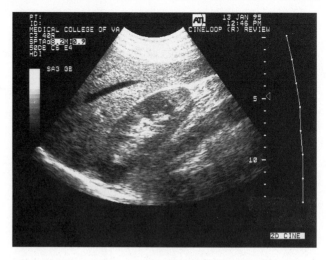

Figure 13-5

12. Why is ultrasonography ideal for examination of the fetus?_____

_____

_____

13. What piece of radiographic equipment is shown in Figure 13-6? _____

_____

_____

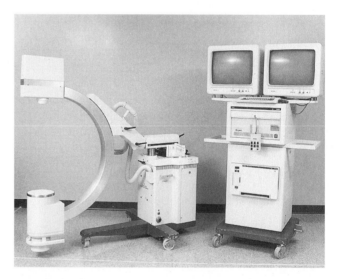

Figure 13-6

14. What is the advantage of fluoroscopy?_____

_____

_____

15. Locate the following structures in the correct abdominal quadrant.

    RUQ = Right Upper Quadrant   LUQ = Left Upper Quadrant

    RLQ = Right Lower Quadrant   LLQ = Left Lower Quadrant

    A. Gallbladder_____   B. Spleen_____

    C. Appendix_____   D. Liver_____

    E. Stomach_____   F. Left Ovary_____

■ Exercise B – Pathology

1. What pathologic condition(s) is/are detected with the use of cholecystography? _____

   _____

   _____

2. What type of examination is necessary to identify a pneumothorax? _____

   _____

   _____

3. What type of examination(s) would a patient experiencing a possible ureteral obstruction undergo to confirm the diagnosis? _____

   _____

   _____

4. What is the one condition that an MIBG scan is useful in diagnosing? _____

   _____

   _____

5. Will pressure readings from a Swan-Ganz catheter placed in the pulmonary artery be useful in diagnosing pulmonary embolism? _____

   _____

   _____

6. What is the purpose of performing a Gram stain? __

   _____

   _____

7. The patient is suspected to have a spinal cord tumor. Will an MRI or a CT scan be more useful in visualizing the soft tissue tumor? _____

   _____

   _____

8. What is considered the first step in determining the etiology of a patient's condition? Why? _____

   _____

   _____

9. Three types of visualization may be used by the examiner during a physical exam. Name the three types, explain how they differ, list any special equipment that may be needed for each, and give at least one example of each type.

   A. _____

   _____

   B. _____

   _____

   C. _____

   _____

10. To confirm a preliminary diagnosis of deep vein thrombosis, what diagnostic examination will be ordered by the physician? _____

    _____

    _____

11. A bone scan is an example of what type of scan? The term *hot spot* refers to what aspect of the scan, and what condition might be indicated by its presence? _____

    _____

    _____

12. Name the two methods of administering radiation therapy. What is the purpose of administering radiation therapy? _____

    _____

    _____

    _____

13. The physician has ordered a blood gas study. Will the blood be drawn from a venous or arterial source? _____

_____

_____

14. What is the normal amount of glucose expected in a urine sample? Use Table 13-3 from the textbook to determine your answer. _____

_____

_____

15. A "culture and sensitivity" has been ordered. The organism has been "cultured" and identified. What is determined by the "sensitivity" portion of the exam?

_____

_____

■ Exercise C – Operation

1. Name the five types of cholecystography.

   A. _____   B. _____

   C. _____   D. _____

   E. _____

2. What purpose does a "scout" film (X-ray) serve?

   _____

   _____

3. Is transesophageal echocardiography an invasive procedure? Why? _____

   _____

   _____

4. What does the term *noninvasive* mean?

   _____

   _____

5. What is the ideal location for insertion of a Swan-Ganz pulmonary artery catheter? List two alternative locations. _____

   _____

   _____

6. List four intraoperative applications for fluoroscopy.

   A. _____

   B. _____

   C. _____

   D. _____

7. Explain the difference(s) between incisional biopsy and excisional biopsy. _____

   _____

   _____

8. The surgeon has requested that fluid aspirated from the thoracic cavity be sent to the laboratory to be cultured for aerobic and anaerobic organisms. What special supplies (if any) will be needed? _____

   _____

   _____

9. The surgeon has requested a frozen section on a piece of breast tissue that has been excised. Will the specimen be placed in formalin? Why?

   _____

   _____

   _____

10. Why is it necessary for the pathologist to be readily available to perform a frozen section?

    _____

    _____

    _____

11. A six-month-old is scheduled to undergo a CT scan with general anesthesia. What is the most likely reason that general anesthesia will be administered? _____

    _____

    _____

12. Explain the difference between a diagnostic and a therapeutic procedure. _____

    _____

    _____

13. List the steps, in order, for percutaneous placement of a femoral artery catheter using the Seldinger technique.

   A. _____

   B. _____

   C. _____

   D. _____

   E. _____

   F. _____

   G. _____

   H. _____

14. What is the difference between a simple voided urine specimen and a clean-catch specimen? What supplies are needed for each? _____

   _____

   _____

   _____

15. Panendoscopy of the upper aerodigestive tract has been scheduled. What structures will be visualized, and what, if any, specialized equipment will be needed? _____

   _____

   _____

■ Exercise D – Specific Variations

Student Name _____ Date _____

Instructor _____

Surgical Procedure – Student Case Study Report

The student will be provided with basic patient information (real or simulated) and is expected to complete the following case study.

1. Procedure name: _____

   _____

   _____

2. Definition of procedure: _____

   _____

   _____

   _____

   _____

3. What is the purpose of the procedure? _____

   _____

   _____

   _____

   _____

4. What is the expected outcome of the procedure?

   _____

   _____

   _____

   _____

5. Patient age: _____

6. Gender: _____

7. Additional pertinent patient information: _____

   _____

   _____

   _____

8. Probable preoperative diagnosis: _____

   _____

   _____

   _____

   _____

9. How was the diagnosis determined? _____

   _____

   _____

   _____

   _____

10. Discuss the relevant anatomy. _____

    _____

    _____

    _____

    _____

    _____

11. List the general and procedure-specific equipment that will be needed for the procedure.

   _____   _____

   _____   _____

   _____   _____

   _____   _____

   _____   _____

   _____   _____

12. List the general and procedure-specific instruments that will be needed for the procedure.

_____   _____

_____   _____

_____   _____

_____   _____

_____   _____

_____   _____

13. List the basic and procedure-specific supplies that will be needed for the procedure.

Pack _____

Basin _____

Gloves _____

Blades _____

Drapes _____

_____

Drains _____

Dressings _____

_____

Suture–Type of Suture, Needle (if applicable), and Anticipated Tissue Usage

_____   _____

_____   _____

_____   _____

_____   _____

_____   _____

Pharmaceuticals

_____   _____

_____   _____

_____   _____

_____   _____

Miscellaneous

_____   _____

_____   _____

_____   _____

_____   _____

_____   _____

14. Operative preparation: _____

_____

_____

_____

_____

_____

15. What type of anesthesia will likely be used? Why?

_____

_____

_____

_____

16. List any special anesthesia equipment that may be needed. _____

_____

_____

_____

_____

_____

17. Patient position during the procedure: _____

_____

_____

_____

_____

18. What supplies will be necessary for positioning?

_____

_____

_____

_____

_____

19. What type of shave/skin preparation will be necessary (if any)?_____

_____

_____

_____

_____

20. Define the anatomic perimeters of the prep.

_____

_____

_____

_____

_____

21. List the order in which the drapes will be applied, and describe any specific variations.

_____

_____

_____

_____

_____

_____

22. List any practical considerations.

_____

_____

_____

_____

_____

_____

23. List the procedural steps, and describe the preparatory and supportive actions of the STSR during each step (use additional space if necessary).

Operative Procedure	Technical Considerations
1.	•
	•
2.	•
	•
3.	•
	•
4.	•
	•
5.	•
	•

Operative Procedure *(continued)*	**Technical Considerations** *(continued)*
6.	•
	•
7.	•
	•
8.	•
	•
9.	•
	•
10.	•
	•

24. What is the postoperative diagnosis?_____

_____

_____

_____

_____

_____

25. Describe the immediate postoperative care.

_____

_____

_____

26. What is the patient's long-term prognosis?

_____

_____

_____

_____

_____

_____

27. What are the possible complications?_____

_____

_____

28. Comments or questions:_____

_____

_____

_____

_____

_____

_____

29. What is the most valuable information you obtained from preparing this surgical procedure case study?

_____

_____

_____

_____

■ Case Studies

□ CASE STUDY 1

Paul, a young athlete, has been scheduled for surgical removal of a Baker's cyst.

1. What is a Baker's cyst?

   _____

   _____

   _____

   _____

2. What diagnostic radiographic exam may have been performed to diagnose Paul's cyst?

   _____

   _____

   _____

   _____

3. In what position will Paul be placed to remove the Baker's cyst?

   _____

   _____

   _____

   _____

   □

☐ CASE STUDY 2

Lynn has just suffered a fall off a stepladder. She fell backwards, striking her head against the wall. She temporarily lost consciousness but is now awake, alert, and oriented. Lynn was transferred to the emergency department at the local hospital by ambulance with a cervical collar in place. She responds appropriately to verbal commands and is able to move all four extremities.

1. Lynn is complaining that the collar is too tight. Should it be removed? Why?

_____

_____

_____

_____

2. What diagnostic examination must be performed prior to removal of the cervical collar?

_____

_____

_____

_____

3. What type of physician specialist will be needed to interpret the results of the diagnostic exam?

_____

_____

_____

_____

_____

☐

General Surgery

OBJECTIVES

After studying this chapter, the reader should be able to:

A 1. Discuss the relevant anatomy and physiology of the abdominal wall, digestive system, hepatic and biliary system, pancreas, spleen, thyroid, and breast.

P 2. Describe the pathology and related terminology of each system or organ that prompts surgical intervention.

3. Discuss any preoperative diagnostic procedures and tests.

4. Discuss any special preoperative preparation procedures related to general surgery procedures.

O 5. Identify the names and uses of general surgery instruments, supplies, and drugs.

6. Identify the names and uses of special equipment related to general surgery.

7. Discuss the intraoperative preparation of the patient undergoing a general surgical procedure.

8. Define and give an overview of illustrative general surgery procedures.

9. Discuss the purpose and expected outcomes of the illustrative procedures.

10. Discuss the immediate postoperative care and possible complications of the illustrative procedures.

S 11. Discuss any specific variations related to the preoperative, intraoperative, and postoperative care of the general surgery patient.

■ Select Key Terms

Define the following:

1. absorption _____

   _____

2. anastomosis _____

   _____

3. ascites _____

   _____

4. bile _____

   _____

5. chole- _____

   _____

6. chyle _____

   _____

7. chyme _____

   _____

8. -cysto _____

   _____

9. -docho- _____

   _____

10. -ectomy _____

    _____

11. excision _____

    _____

12. incision _____

    _____

13. lysis _____

    _____

14. necrosis _____

    _____

15. -oma _____

    _____

16. -ostomy _____

    _____

17. -otomy _____

    _____

18. parietal _____

    _____

19. peristalsis _____

    _____

20. peritoneum _____

    _____

21. portal venous system _____

    _____

22. -stasis _____

    _____

23. stenosis _____

    _____

24. ulcer _____

    _____

25. viscera _____

    _____

■ Exercise A – Anatomy

1. Trace the alimentary pathway by placing the following elements in the correct order.

A. _____ Anus

B. _____ Ascending colon

C. _____ Body of stomach

D. _____ Cardia of stomach

E. _____ Cardiac sphincter

F. _____ Cecum

G. _____ Descending colon

H. _____ Duodenum

I. _____ Epiglottis

J. _____ Esophagus

K. _____ Fundus of stomach

L. _____ Hepatic flexure

M. _____ Ileocecal valve

N. _____ Ileum

O. _____ Jejunum

P. _____ Labia

Q. _____ Mouth

R. _____ Pharynx

S. _____ Pyloric sphincter

T. _____ Pylorus of stomach

U. _____ Rectum

V. _____ Sigmoid colon

W. _____ Splenic flexure

X. _____ Transverse colon

Y. _____ Uvula

2. Identify the accessory digestive ducts and organs shown in Figure 14-1.

A. _____   B. _____

C. _____   D. _____

E. _____   F. _____

G. _____   H. _____

I. _____   J. _____

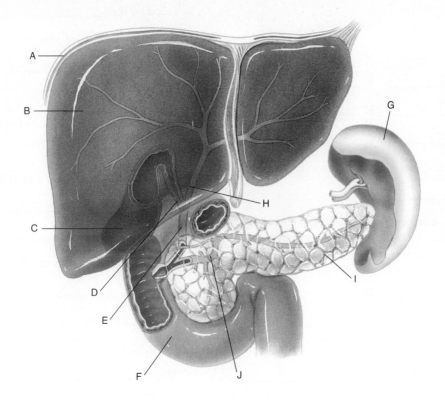

Figure 14-1

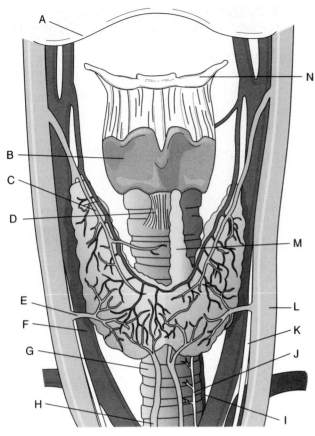

Figure 14-2

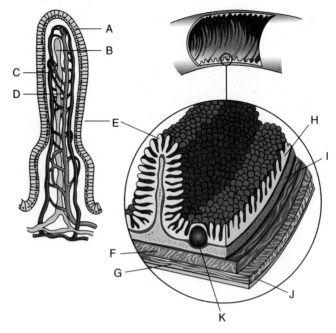

Figure 14-3

3. Identify the structures of the thyroid gland shown in Figure 14-2.

A. _____   B. _____

C. _____   D. _____

E. _____   F. _____

G. _____   H. _____

I. _____   J. _____

K. _____   L. _____

M. _____   N. _____

4. Identify the components of the intestinal wall shown in Figure 14-3.

A. _____   B. _____

C. _____   D. _____

E. _____   F. _____

G. _____   H. _____

I. _____   J. _____

K. _____

5. The gallbladder is located in the _____ _____ quadrant of the abdomen.

6. Linea alba literally means _____ _____ and will be found in the _____ abdominal wall.

7. Parasympathetic innervation to the stomach is provided by the _____ nerve.

8. The four layers of the wall of the colon are _____, _____, _____, and _____.

9. The pancreas is classified as both a(n) _____ and _____ gland.

10. What is the primary function of the peritoneum?

_____

_____

11. Name the five sections of the stomach.

A. _____

B. _____

C. _____

D. _____

E. _____

12. Where are the islets of Langerhans located, and what is their function? _____

_____

_____

13. What is the largest organ in the normal abdominal cavity? _____

_____

14. List the functions that are performed by the cells of the liver.

A. _____

B. _____

C. _____

D. _____

E. _____

F. _____

15. What is the function of the sphincter of Oddi?

_____

_____

■ Exercise B – Pathology

1. Peptic ulcers are most frequently found in which location? _____

_____

_____

2. Explain the difference between an incarcerated and a strangulated hernia. _____

_____

_____

3. Is a direct hernia congenital or acquired?_____

_____

_____

4. What is diverticulitis?_____

_____

_____

5. What causes intra-abdominal adhesions? _____

_____

_____

6. Are a hemorrhoid and a pile the same? _____

_____

_____

7. What are the two types of choleliths, and what is the composition of each?

A. _____

B. _____

8. What is "referred" pain? _____

_____

_____

9. What is the usual cause of appendicitis? _____

_____

10. Thrombocytopenia is a deficiency of _____ in the blood.

11. Which diagnostic tools will be useful in determining liver pathology? _____

_____

_____

12. List four of the causes of varicose veins of the lower extremity.

A. _____

B. _____

C. _____

D. _____

13. Define gynecomastia, and describe the surgical treatment that may be recommended to treat the condition. _____

_____

_____

14. Overactivity of the thyroid gland is referred to as

_____

15. What is meant by the term *staging* in reference to malignant tumors?_____

_____

_____

■ Exercise C – Operation

1. Laparoscopic Nissen fundoplication is performed to treat which condition(s)? _____

_____

_____

2. What structure is dilated with a Maloney dilator? Is the Maloney dilator inserted under sterile conditions? Why? _____

_____

_____

3. List two reasons for performing a gastrostomy.

    A._____

    B._____

4. Explain what is meant by the phrase "mobilize the bowel."

    _____

    _____

5. List the three basic configurations for intestinal anastomosis.

    A._____

    B._____

    C._____

6. Describe the technique used to care for instrumentation and supplies that have been exposed to the inside of the intestinal tract.

    _____

    _____

7. What is a stoma? _____

    _____

    _____

8. What is the purpose of a T-tube, and where is it placed? _____

_____

_____

9. Why is it important to expel all air from the cholangiogram system prior to an intraoperative cholangiogram? _____

_____

_____

10. What is the reason for providing a second setup to perform a breast reconstruction following a modified radical mastectomy due to a malignancy? _____

_____

_____

11. Why is it important for the STSR to maintain the sterile field until the patient is extubated and breathing freely following a thyroidectomy?

_____

_____

12. What instruments and supplies will be needed to enter the common bile duct for CBDE? _____

13. Name the two positions that provide access to the anus.

    A._____

    B._____

14. What type of procedure is performed through a McBurney's incision?_____

_____

_____

15. McVay repair is performed to correct which condition?_____

_____

■ Exercise D – Specific Variations

Student Name _____ Date _____

Instructor _____

Surgical Procedure – Student Case Study Report

The student will be provided with basic patient information (real or simulated) and is expected to complete the following case study.

1. Procedure name: _____

   _____

   _____

2. Definition of procedure: _____

   _____

   _____

   _____

3. What is the purpose of the procedure?_____

   _____

   _____

   _____

4. What is the expected outcome of the procedure?

   _____

   _____

   _____

   _____

5. Patient age:_____

6. Gender:_____

7. Additional pertinent patient information: _____

   _____

   _____

   _____

8. Probable preoperative diagnosis: _____

   _____

   _____

   _____

   _____

9. How was the diagnosis determined?_____

   _____

   _____

   _____

   _____

10. Discuss the relevant anatomy. _____

    _____

    _____

    _____

    _____

    _____

11. List the general and procedure-specific equipment that will be needed for the procedure.

    _____   _____

    _____   _____

    _____   _____

    _____   _____

    _____   _____

    _____   _____

12. List the general and procedure-specific instruments that will be needed for the procedure.

_____   _____

_____   _____

_____   _____

_____   _____

_____   _____

_____   _____

13. List the basic and procedure-specific supplies that will be needed for the procedure.

Pack _____

Basin _____

Gloves _____

Blades _____

Drapes _____

_____

Drains _____

Dressings _____

_____

Suture—Type of Suture, Needle (if applicable), and Anticipated Tissue Usage

_____   _____

_____   _____

_____   _____

_____   _____

_____   _____

_____   _____

Pharmaceuticals

_____   _____

_____   _____

_____   _____

_____   _____

_____   _____

Miscellaneous

_____   _____

_____   _____

_____   _____

_____   _____

_____   _____

_____   _____

14. Operative preparation: _____

_____

_____

_____

_____

_____

15. What type of anesthesia will likely be used? Why?

_____

_____

_____

_____

16. List any special anesthesia equipment that may be needed. _____

_____

_____

_____

_____

17. Patient position during the procedure: _____

_____

_____

18. What supplies will be necessary for positioning?

_____

_____

_____

_____

_____

19. What type of shave/skin preparation will be necessary (if any)?_____

_____

_____

_____

_____

20. Define the anatomic perimeters of the prep.

_____

_____

_____

_____

_____

21. List the order in which the drapes will be applied, and describe any specific variations.

_____

_____

_____

_____

_____

_____

22. List any practical considerations.

_____

_____

_____

_____

_____

23. List the procedural steps, and describe the preparatory and supportive actions of the STSR during each step (use additional space if necessary).

Operative Procedure	Technical Considerations
1.	•
	•
2.	•
	•
3.	•
	•
4.	•
	•
5.	•
	•

(continues)

Operative Procedure *(continued)*	**Technical Considerations** *(continued)*
6.	•
	•
7.	•
	•
8.	•
	•
9.	•
	•
10.	•
	•

24. What is the postoperative diagnosis? _____

_____

_____

_____

_____

25. Describe the immediate postoperative care.

_____

_____

_____

_____

_____

_____

26. What is the patient's long-term prognosis?

_____

_____

_____

_____

_____

27. What are the possible complications? _____

_____

_____

_____

_____

_____

_____

28. Comments or questions: _____

_____

_____

_____

_____

_____

_____

29. What is the most valuable information you obtained from preparing this surgical procedure case study?

_____

_____

_____

_____

■ Case Studies

□ CASE STUDY 1

Lin Su is a 21-year-old female college student. She was admitted to the college's health center for right lower quadrant pain, nausea, and low-grade fever. She was diagnosed with acute appendicitis, and surgery was scheduled.

1. What causes appendicitis?

   _____

   _____

   _____

   _____

2. What are the signs and symptoms of appendicitis?

   _____

   _____

   _____

   _____

3. Describe a McBurney's incision.

   _____

   _____

   _____

   _____

4. What is the primary difference between a McBurney's and a Rockey-Davis incision?

   _____

   _____

   _____

   _____

□ CASE STUDY 2

Jon and Linda are both 41-year-old computer programmers. They are in the preoperative holding area. Each is scheduled for a hernia repair in the groin area.

1. What are the chances that Jon's hernia is a femoral hernia?

   _____

   _____

   _____

   _____

2. Jon's hernia is said to be incarcerated. What does this mean?

   _____

   _____

   _____

   _____

3. If Linda has a femoral hernia, the hernia exists below what anatomical marker?

   _____

   _____

   _____

   _____

4. Describe Hesselbach's triangle.

   _____

   _____

   _____

   _____

5. Jon's hernia was described in the postoperative report as a direct hernia. Is it probable that the hernia was congenital in nature?

   _____

   _____

   _____

   _____

CHAPTER 15

Obstetric and Gynecologic Surgery

OBJECTIVES

After studying this chapter, the reader should be able to:

A 1. Discuss the relevant anatomy and physiology of the female reproductive system.

P 2. Describe the pathology of the female reproductive system that prompts surgical intervention and the related terminology.

3. Discuss any special preoperative obstetric and gynecologic diagnostic procedures/tests.

O 4. Discuss any special preoperative preparation procedures related to obstetric/gynecologic procedures.

5. Identify the names and uses of obstetric and gynecologic instruments, supplies, and drugs.

6. Identify the names and uses of special equipment related to obstetric/gynecologic surgery.

7. Discuss the intraoperative preparation of the patient undergoing an obstetric or gynecologic procedure.

8. Define and give an overview of the obstetric/gynecologic procedure.

9. Discuss the purpose and expected outcomes of the obstetric/gynecologic procedure.

10. Discuss the immediate postoperative care and possible complications of the obstetric/gynecologic procedure.

S 11. Discuss any specific variations related to the preoperative, intraoperative, and postoperative care of the obstetric/gynecologic patient.

■ Select Key Terms

Define the following:

1. adnexa _____

_____

2. bony pelvis _____

_____

3. breech _____

_____

4. cesarean section _____

_____

5. corpus luteum _____

_____

6. CPD _____

_____

7. curettage _____

_____

8. delivery forceps _____

_____

9. DUB _____

_____

10. dystocia _____

_____

11. episiotomy _____

_____

12. exenteration _____

_____

13. fimbria _____

_____

14. fistula _____

_____

15. gravida _____

_____

16. LEEP _____

_____

17. ligament _____

_____

18. marsupialization _____

_____

19. myoma _____

_____

20. occiput anterior _____

_____

21. parity _____

_____

22. perineum _____

_____

23. Pfannenstiel _____

_____

24. vestibule _____

_____

■ Exercise A – Anatomy

1. Identify the structures of the external female genitalia shown in Figure 15-1.

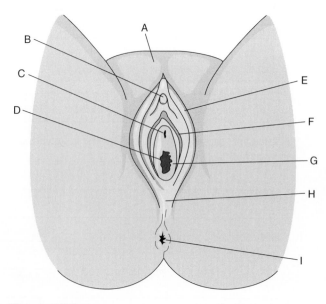

Figure 15-1

A._____

B._____

C._____

D._____

E._____

F._____

G._____

H._____

I._____

2. Identify the structures shown in Figure 15-2.

A._____

B._____

C._____

D._____

E._____

F._____

G._____

H._____

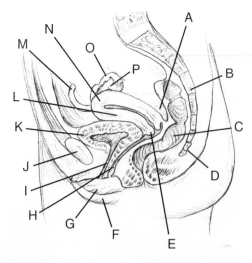

Figure 15-2

I._____

J._____

K._____

L._____

M._____

N._____

O._____

P._____

3. Identify the structures of the female reproductive system shown in Figure 15-3.

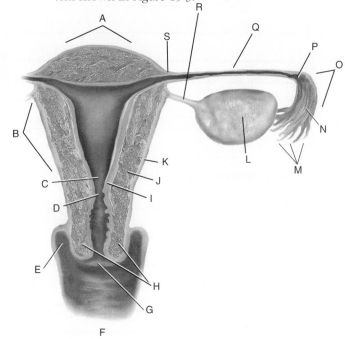

Figure 15-3

A. _____

B. _____

C. _____

D._____

E. _____

F. _____

G._____

H._____

I. _____

J. _____

K._____

L. _____

M._____

N._____

O._____

P. _____

Q._____

R. _____

S. _____

4. What is the fornix?_____

_____

_____

5. Describe the locations of the internal and external cervical os. _____

_____

_____

6. List the three layers of the uterine wall.

A. _____

B. _____

C. _____

7. Where are the Bartholin's glands located? What is their function? _____

_____

_____

8. List the structures contained within the broad ligament.

A. _____

B. _____

C. _____

D._____

E. _____

F. _____

9. What are the other two names for the fallopian tubes?

_____

_____

_____

10. Describe the location of the ovaries. _____

_____

_____

11. Name the two hormones from the anterior pituitary that stimulate the ovarian cycle. _____

_____

_____

12. Name the two hormones that are produced by the ovary. _____

_____

_____

13. Name the bones of the pelvic girdle. _____

_____

_____

14. What is the main muscle of the pelvic floor? Name its three components. _____

_____

A. _____

B. _____

C. _____

15. Branches of which nerve provide sensation to the perineum?_____

_____

_____

■ Exercise B – Pathology

1. Are Braxton Hicks contractions an indication that delivery of the fetus is imminent? _____

2. Cord blood is collected routinely with every delivery. Why? _____

3. What does "fetal distress" mean? _____

4. What is the most common reason for performing a cesarean section? _____

5. Define *cystocele*, and give two reasons why a cystocele may occur. _____

6. What condition is diagnosed with the use of the Pap smear? _____

7. List the possible sites for ectopic pregnancy.

8. What is meant by the term *incompetent cervix*? What procedure is performed to treat the condition during pregnancy? _____

9. Define *leiomyoma*. _____

10. What are the symptoms of endometriosis? _____

11. Is ultrasound useful in diagnosing a malignancy?

12. What is the most common symptom of uterine cancer? _____

13. List two placental conditions that may necessitate a cesarean section. _____

14. Amenorrhea is the condition of _____.

15. What is a pedunculated lesion? _____

■ Exercise C – Operation

1. In what position will the patient be placed to accomplish a D&C? In addition to the basic position, which position may be used to enhance the surgeon's view of the anatomy? _____

2. Explain the usefulness of the Trendelenburg position during pelvic surgery. _____

3. Describe the complications that the patient may suffer from an undiagnosed or improperly closed perineal laceration. _____

4. Name two types of suction devices that may be used to clear a neonate's airway. _____

_____

_____

5. What are the advantages to a "classic" approach for a cesarean section? _____

_____

_____

6. Name the three approaches that are available for tubal sterilization.

    A. _____

    B. _____

    C. _____

7. Posterior colporrhaphy is performed to treat which condition? _____

_____

_____

8. What is Lugol's solution used for? _____

_____

_____

9. What are some advantages to LAVH? _____

_____

_____

10. What is the importance of draining the bladder prior to D&C? _____

_____

_____

11. Why is a Foley catheter placed prior to a cesarean section? _____

_____

_____

12. List the structures that will be removed during total pelvic exenteration. _____

_____

_____

13. What safety measures must be implemented when a laser is in use? _____

_____

_____

14. List the drape components that are necessary to drape a patient in the lithotomy position. Describe the draping sequence. _____

_____

_____

15. What structure(s) is/are removed during a TAH? ___

_____

_____

■ Exercise D – Specific Variations

Student Name _____ Date _____

Instructor _____

Surgical Procedure – Student Case Study Report

The student will be provided with basic patient information (real or simulated) and is expected to complete the following case study.

1. Procedure name: _____

   _____

   _____

2. Definition of procedure: _____

   _____

   _____

   _____

3. What is the purpose of the procedure? _____

   _____

   _____

   _____

   _____

4. What is the expected outcome of the procedure?

   _____

   _____

   _____

   _____

5. Patient age: _____

6. Gender: _____

7. Additional pertinent patient information: _____

   _____

   _____

   _____

8. Probable preoperative diagnosis: _____

   _____

   _____

   _____

   _____

   _____

9. How was the diagnosis determined? _____

   _____

   _____

   _____

   _____

   _____

10. Discuss the relevant anatomy. _____

    _____

    _____

    _____

    _____

11. List the general and procedure-specific equipment that will be needed for the procedure.

    _____   _____

    _____   _____

    _____   _____

    _____   _____

    _____   _____

12. List the general and procedure-specific instruments that will be needed for the procedure.

_____ _____

_____ _____

_____ _____

_____ _____

_____ _____

_____ _____

13. List the basic and procedure-specific supplies that will be needed for the procedure.

Pack _____

Basin _____

Gloves _____

Blades _____

Drapes _____

_____

Drains _____

Dressings _____

_____

Suture—Type of Suture, Needle (if applicable), and Anticipated Tissue Usage

_____ _____

_____ _____

_____ _____

_____ _____

_____ _____

_____ _____

Pharmaceuticals

_____ _____

_____ _____

_____ _____

_____ _____

_____ _____

Miscellaneous

_____ _____

_____ _____

_____ _____

_____ _____

_____ _____

_____ _____

14. Operative preparation: _____

_____

_____

_____

_____

_____

15. What type of anesthesia will likely be used? Why?

_____

_____

_____

_____

_____

16. List any special anesthesia equipment that may be needed. _____

_____

_____

_____

_____

_____

_____

17. Patient position during the procedure: _____

_____

_____

_____

_____

18. What supplies will be necessary for positioning?

_____

_____

_____

_____

_____

19. What type of shave/skin preparation will be necessary (if any)? _____

_____

_____

_____

_____

20. Define the anatomic perimeters of the prep.

_____

_____

_____

_____

_____

21. List the order in which the drapes will be applied, and describe any specific variations.

_____

_____

_____

_____

_____

_____

_____

_____

22. List any practical considerations.

_____

_____

_____

_____

_____

_____

23. List the procedural steps, and describe the preparatory and supportive actions of the STSR during each step (use additional space if necessary).

Operative Procedure	Technical Considerations
1.	•
	•
2.	•
	•
3.	•
	•
4.	•
	•
5.	•
	•

(continues)

Operative Procedure *(continued)*	Technical Considerations *(continued)*
6.	•
	•
7.	•
	•
8.	•
	•
9.	•
	•
10.	•
	•

24. What is the postoperative diagnosis? _____

_____

_____

_____

_____

_____

25. Describe the immediate postoperative care.

_____

_____

_____

_____

_____

26. What is the patient's long-term prognosis?

_____

_____

_____

_____

_____

_____

27. What are the possible complications? _____

_____

_____

_____

_____

_____

28. Comments or questions: _____

_____

_____

_____

_____

_____

29. What is the most valuable information you obtained from preparing this surgical procedure case study?

_____

_____

_____

■ Case Studies

□ CASE STUDY 1

Shannon is a 23-year-old primipara who has just been admitted to the labor and delivery unit. She has had a normal pregnancy, and sonograms confirm only one fetus. Her cervix is dilated to 4 cm.

1. How long, on average, would you expect her labor to continue?

_____

_____

_____

_____

2. To what does the term *presentation* refer?

_____

_____

_____

_____

3. To what does the term *position* refer?

_____

_____

_____

_____

4. To what does the term *station* refer?

_____

_____

_____

_____

☐ CASE STUDY 2

Correta has been admitted for a diagnostic laparoscopy for pelvic pain of unknown origin.

1. What equipment will be needed for the procedure?

    _____

    _____

    _____

    _____

2. What instruments will be needed for the procedure?

    _____

    _____

    _____

    _____

3. In what position will Correta be placed?

    _____

    _____

    _____

    _____

4. What are the common complications of laparoscopy?

    _____

    _____

    _____

    _____

    ☐

CHAPTER 16

Ophthalmic Surgery

OBJECTIVES

After studying this chapter, the reader should be able to:

A 1. Discuss the anatomy of the eye.

P 2. Describe the pathology that prompts surgical intervention of the eye and related terminology.

   3. Discuss any special preoperative ophthalmic diagnostic procedures/tests.

O 4. Discuss any special preoperative preparation procedures.

   5. Identify the names and uses of ophthalmic instruments, supplies, and drugs.

   6. Identify the names and uses of special equipment.

   7. Discuss the intraoperative preparation of the patient undergoing an ophthalmic procedure.

   8. Define and give an overview of the ophthalmic procedure.

   9. Discuss the purpose and expected outcomes of the ophthalmic procedures.

  10. Discuss the immediate postoperative care and possible complications of the ophthalmic procedures.

S 11. Discuss any specific variations related to the preoperative, intraoperative, and postoperative care of the ophthalmic patient.

■ Select Key Terms

Define the following:

1. anterior chamber _____

   _____

2. BSS _____

   _____

3. cataract _____

   _____

4. chalazion _____

   _____

5. dacryo- _____

   _____

6. diathermy _____

   _____

7. enucleation _____

   _____

8. extracapsular cataract extraction _____

   _____

9. extrinsic muscles _____

   _____

10. globe _____

    _____

11. intracapsular cataract extraction _____

    _____

12. iridotomy _____

    _____

13. kerato- _____

    _____

14. lacrimal _____

    _____

15. ocutome _____

    _____

16. posterior chamber _____

    _____

17. retrobulbar _____

    _____

18. strabismus _____

    _____

19. trephine _____

    _____

20. tunic _____

    _____

■ Exercise A – Anatomy

1. Identify the structures of the eye shown in Figure 16-1.

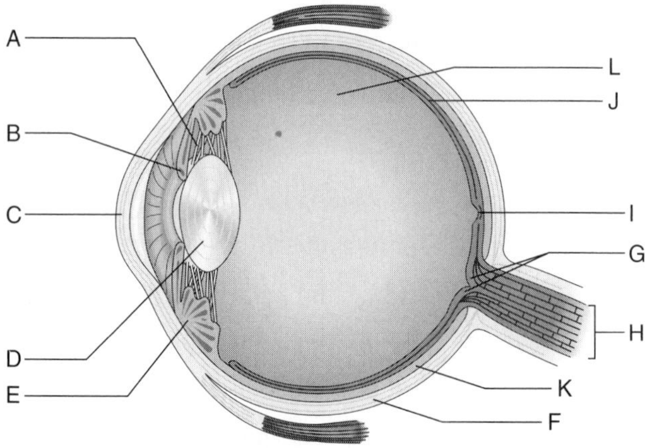

Figure 16-1

A. _____

B. _____

C. _____

D. _____

E. _____

F. _____

G. _____

H. _____

I. _____

J. _____

K. _____

L. _____

2. Identify the nerves of the eye shown in Figure 16-2.

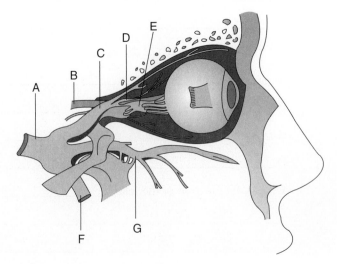

Figure 16-2

A. _____

B. _____

C. _____

D. _____

E. _____

F. _____

G. _____

3. Identify the muscles of the eye shown in Figure 16-3.

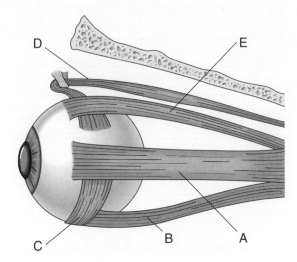

Figure 16-3

A. _____

B. _____

C. _____

D. _____

E. _____

4. Identify the structures of the lacrimal apparatus shown in Figure 16-4.

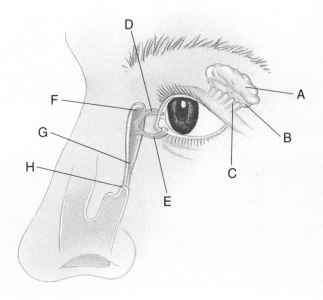

Figure 16-4

A. _____

B. _____

C. _____

D. _____

E. _____

F. _____

G. _____

H. _____

5. Name the three tunics of the eye.

A. _____

B. _____

C. _____

6. Name the two intrinsic muscles of the eye.

   A. _____

   B. _____

7. Name the bones that form the orbit.

   A. _____

   B. _____

   C. _____

   D. _____

   E. _____

   F. _____

   G. _____

8. Name the six extrinsic muscles of the eye and the primary function of each.

   A. _____

   B. _____

   C. _____

   D. _____

   E. _____

   F. _____

9. What are the four tissue layers that make up the cornea?

   A. _____

   B. _____

   C. _____

   D. _____

10. _____ humor fills the posterior chamber of the eye.

11. Briefly explain the process of accommodation.

   _____

   _____

   _____

   _____

12. Describe the location of the crystalline lens.

   _____

   _____

   _____

   _____

13. List the refractive media of the eye.

   A. _____

   B. _____

   C. _____

   D. _____

14. What is the function of the iris? _____

   _____

   _____

   _____

   _____

15. Describe the functions of the rods and the cones.

   _____

   _____

   _____

   _____

■ Exercise B – Pathology

1. Give three reasons for cataract formation.

   A. _____

   B. _____

   C. _____

2. Why is a cataract considered a condition rather than a disease? _____

   _____

   _____

   _____

3. Describe what happens when a retinal detachment occurs. _____

_____

_____

_____

_____

4. Explain why a patient may see "spots" or "flashes of light" with the development of a retinal detachment.

_____

_____

_____

_____

5. What is a chalazion? _____

_____

_____

_____

_____

6. Explain the difference between comitant and in-comitant strabismus. _____

_____

_____

_____

_____

7. List four causes of corneal clouding.

A. _____

B. _____

C. _____

D. _____

8. Name and describe the visual defect shown in Figure 16-5.

_____

_____

_____

_____

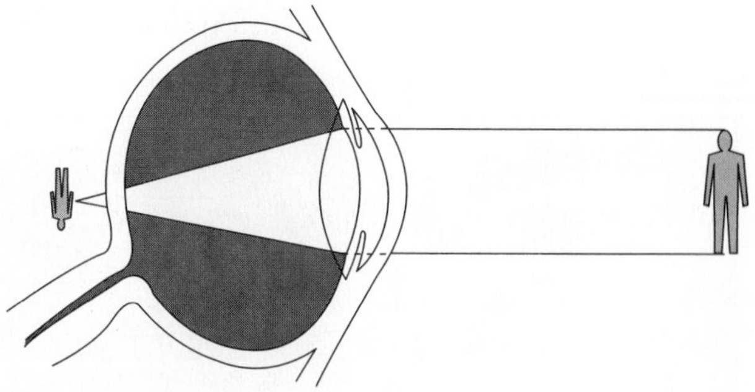

Figure 16-5

9. Name and describe the visual defect shown in Figure 16-6.

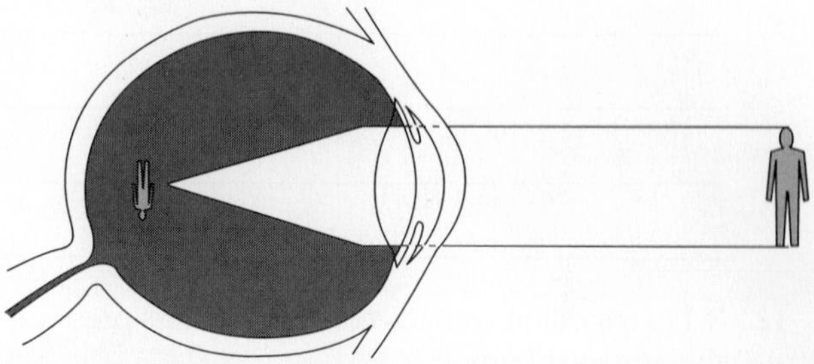

Figure 16-6

_____

_____

_____

_____

_____

10. Name and describe the visual defect shown in Figure 16-7.

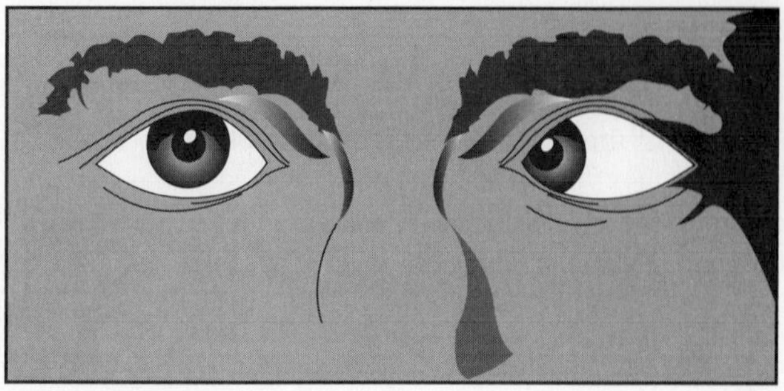

Figure 16-7

_____

_____

_____

_____

11. Name and describe the visual defect shown in Figure 16-8.

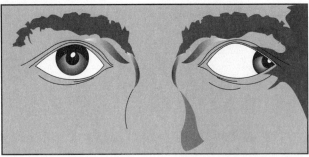

Figure 16-8

_____

_____

_____

_____

12. What condition is characterized by excess pressure of the aqueous humor? _____

_____

_____

_____

_____

13. What is an epiretinal membrane? _____

_____

_____

_____

_____

14. List three indications for enucleation.

A. _____

B. _____

C. _____

15. What visual deficit will occur in a person who lacks cones in the retina? _____

_____

_____

_____

_____

■ Exercise C – Operation

1. How is intraocular pressure measured from within the sterile field? _____

_____

_____

_____

_____

2. What procedure is performed to open the blocked tear ducts of an infant? _____

_____

_____

_____

_____

3. List three methods for cataract extraction.

A. _____

B. _____

C. _____

4. What is a diathermy apparatus used to accomplish?

_____

_____

_____

_____

5. How is cryotherapy used to treat retinal detachment?

_____

_____

_____

_____

6. Recession/resection is used for correcting what condition of the eye? _____

_____

_____

_____

_____

7. What type of instrument is a trephine? In eye surgery, what is it used for? _____

_____

_____

_____

8. What is the purpose of inserting a scleral buckle to treat retinal detachment?_____

_____

_____

_____

9. List four complications that may arise following a scleral buckle procedure.

A._____

B._____

C._____

D._____

10. The topical anesthetic cocaine is often used to prepare the nose for dacryocystorhinostomy, even if a general anesthetic is planned. Why?

_____

_____

_____

_____

11. What is the main advantage of evisceration of the eye over enucleation?

_____

_____

_____

_____

12. What is sodium hyaluronate used for?

_____

_____

_____

13. List the drapes necessary for surgery to expose the eye, and their order of application.

_____

_____

_____

_____

14. What is the purpose of applying fluorescein to the cornea? What tool must be used in conjunction with fluorescein?

_____

_____

_____

_____

15. What is the main advantage of phacoemulsification over traditional extracapsular cataract extraction?

_____

_____

_____

■ Exercise D – Specific Variations

Student Name _____ Date _____

Instructor _____

Surgical Procedure – Student Case Study Report

The student will be provided with basic patient information (real or simulated) and is expected to complete the following case study.

1. Procedure name: _____

_____

_____

2. Definition of procedure: _____

_____

_____

_____

_____

3. What is the purpose of the procedure? _____

_____

_____

_____

4. What is the expected outcome of the procedure?

_____

_____

_____

_____

5. Patient age: _____

6. Gender: _____

7. Additional pertinent patient information: _____

_____

_____

_____

8. Probable preoperative diagnosis: _____

_____

_____

_____

_____

_____

9. How was the diagnosis determined? _____

_____

_____

_____

_____

10. Discuss the relevant anatomy. _____

_____

_____

_____

_____

_____

11. List the general and procedure-specific equipment that will be needed for the procedure.

_____   _____

_____   _____

_____   _____

_____   _____

_____   _____

12. List the general and procedure-specific instruments that will be needed for the procedure.

_____   _____

_____   _____

_____   _____

_____   _____

_____   _____

_____   _____

13. List the basic and procedure-specific supplies that will be needed for the procedure.

Pack _____

Basin _____

Gloves _____

Blades _____

Drapes _____

_____

Drains _____

Dressings _____

_____

Suture—Type of Suture, Needle (if applicable), and Anticipated Tissue Usage

_____   _____

_____   _____

_____   _____

_____   _____

_____   _____

_____   _____

Pharmaceuticals

_____   _____

_____   _____

_____   _____

_____   _____

Miscellaneous

_____   _____

_____   _____

_____   _____

_____   _____

_____   _____

_____   _____

14. Operative preparation: _____

_____

_____

_____

_____

_____

15. What type of anesthesia will likely be used? Why?

_____

_____

_____

_____

_____

16. List any special anesthesia equipment that may be needed. _____

_____

_____

_____

_____

_____

17. Patient position during the procedure: _____

_____

_____

_____

18. What supplies will be necessary for positioning?

_____

_____

_____

_____

_____

19. What type of shave/skin preparation will be necessary (if any)?_____

_____

_____

_____

_____

20. Define the anatomic perimeters of the prep.

_____

_____

_____

_____

_____

_____

21. List the order in which the drapes will be applied, and describe any specific variations.

_____

_____

_____

_____

_____

_____

22. List any practical considerations.

_____

_____

_____

_____

_____

_____

23. List the procedural steps, and describe the preparatory and supportive actions of the STSR during each step (use additional space if necessary).

Operative Procedure	Technical Considerations
1.	•
	•
2.	•
	•
3.	•
	•
4.	•
	•
5.	•
	•

Operative Procedure *(continued)*	Technical Considerations *(continued)*
6.	•
	•
7.	•
	•
8.	•
	•
9.	•
	•
10.	•
	•

24. What is the postoperative diagnosis? _____

_____

_____

_____

_____

25. Describe the immediate postoperative care.

_____

_____

_____

_____

_____

26. What is the patient's long-term prognosis?

_____

_____

_____

_____

27. What are the possible complications? _____

_____

_____

_____

_____

_____

28. Comments or questions: _____

_____

_____

_____

_____

_____

29. What is the most valuable information you obtained from preparing this surgical procedure case study? _____

_____

_____

_____

_____

■ Case Studies

□ CASE STUDY 1

Susan is admitted to the hospital for eye surgery. She was diagnosed in childhood with diabetes and is now 50 years old. Susan also has been diagnosed with retinopathy, a frequent occurrence in diabetic patients. Her vision has been deteriorating over the last several years. She has recently suffered a vitreous hemorrhage due to neovascularization of the eye, which is common in diabetic patients.

1. What procedure will be performed to resolve the problem?

     _____

     _____

     _____

     _____

2. Briefly describe the procedure, and explain how Susan will benefit.

     _____

     _____

     _____

     _____

3. What are the two possible approaches the surgeon may use to enter the eye? Which is preferred?

     _____

     _____

     _____

     _____

4. What piece of equipment is crucial to a vitrectomy?

     _____

     _____

     _____

     _____

5. What substance, if any, will be used to replace the vitreous humor?

     _____

     _____

     _____

     _____

☐ CASE STUDY 2

Ronald has been having trouble with his stereoscopic vision. His wife says that he appears to have a "lazy eye." The amount of misalignment seems to stay the same no matter which direction his eyes are looking. Ronald has been admitted to the ambulatory care center for surgery.

1. What is the correct term for the condition that Ronald has?

2. Would this condition be considered "comitant" or "incomitant?"

3. What surgical procedure will be performed to correct this condition?

4. In which position will Ronald be placed for this procedure?

5. What are the anatomic boundaries for the prep?

Otorhinolaryngologic Surgery

CHAPTER 17

OBJECTIVES

After studying this chapter, the reader should be able to:

A 1. Discuss the relevant anatomy of the ear, nose, and upper aerodigestive tract.

P 2. Describe the pathology that prompts otorhinolaryngologic surgical intervention and the related terminology.

3. Discuss any special preoperative otorhinolaryngologic diagnostic procedures/tests.

O 4. Discuss any special otorhinolaryngologic preoperative preparation procedures.

5. Identify the names and uses of otorhinolaryngologic instruments, supplies, and drugs.

6. Identify the names and uses of special otorhinolaryngologic equipment.

7. Discuss the intraoperative preparation of the patient undergoing an otorhinolaryngologic procedure.

8. Define and give an overview of the otorhinolaryngologic procedures.

9. Discuss the purpose and expected outcomes of the otorhinolaryngologic procedures.

10. Discuss the immediate postoperative care and possible complications of the otorhinolaryngologic procedures.

S 11. Discuss any specific variations related to the preoperative, intraoperative, and postoperative care of the otorhinolaryngologic patient.

■ Select Key Terms

Define the following:

1. aerodigestive tract _____

2. apnea _____

3. carina _____

4. cholesteatoma _____

5. congenital _____

6. dynamic equilibrium _____

7. epiglottis _____

8. epistaxis _____

9. Gelfoam _____

10. glottis _____

11. hydrops _____

12. hypertrophy _____

13. laryngo- _____

14. myringo- _____

15. olfaction _____

16. oropharynx _____

17. oto- _____

18. pharyngotympanic tube _____

19. polyp _____

20. polysomnography _____

21. rhino- _____

22. -sclerosis _____

23. SMR _____

24. T&A _____

25. UPPP _____

■ **Exercise A – Anatomy**

1. Identify the structures of the ear shown in Figure 17-1.

   A. _____ B. _____

   C. _____ D. _____

   E. _____ F. _____

   G. _____ H. _____

2. Identify the structures of the upper aerodigestive tract shown in Figure 17-2.

   A. _____ B. _____

   C. _____ D. _____

   E. _____ F. _____

   G. _____ H. _____

   I. _____ J. _____

   K. _____ L. _____

   M. _____ N. _____

   O. _____ P. _____

   Q. _____

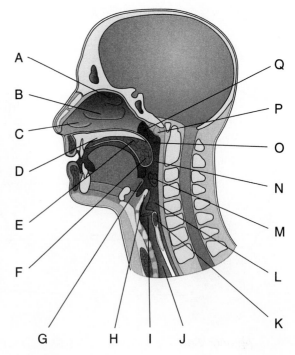

Figure 17-2

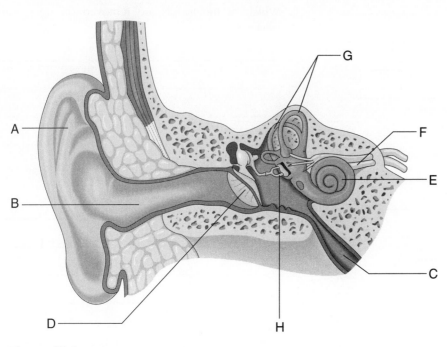

Figure 17-1

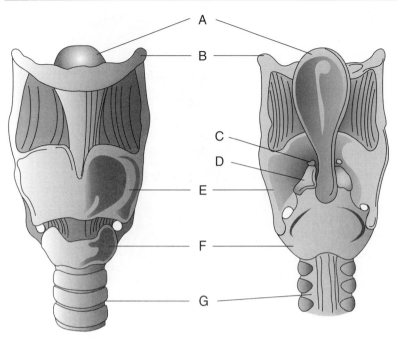

Anterior View   Posterior View   **Figure 17-3**

3. Identify the structures shown in Figure 17-3.

    A._____

    B._____

    C._____

    D._____

    E._____

    F._____

    G._____

4. List two functions of the nose.

    A._____

    _____

    B._____

    _____

5. Which bone houses the mastoid sinus? _____

    _____

    _____

    _____

6. Name the three sections of the pharynx. _____

    A._____

    B._____

    C._____

7. Which of the tonsils are removed during a tonsillectomy? _____

    _____

    _____

    _____

    _____

8. Name the four pairs of paranasal sinuses, and give their locations.

    A._____

    B._____

    C._____

    D._____

9. How many layers comprise the tympanic membrane, and what is the composition of each layer?

_____

_____

_____

_____

10. Where would you find the umbo and cone of light, and what are they? _____

_____

_____

_____

11. Provide the scientific and common names for the ossicles in their proper sequence, moving from lateral to medial. _____

_____

_____

_____

12. How many nasal bones does each individual normally have, and what is their function? _____

_____

_____

_____

13. What are nasal conchae? Describe their function.

_____

_____

_____

14. What is the main source of arterial blood to the nose, and from which vessel is it derived?

_____

_____

_____

15. Where are the adenoids located?_____

_____

_____

_____

_____

■ Exercise B – Pathology

1. Can tonsillitis affect the palatine tonsils? _____

_____

_____

_____

_____

2. Which nerve is affected in a patient with sensorineural deafness? _____

_____

_____

3. What is the cause of hypertrophied turbinates?

_____

_____

_____

4. What is the cause of obstructive sleep apnea?

_____

_____

_____

_____

5. What is the most common cause of otitis media?

_____

_____

_____

6. What causes the nasal septum to deviate from the midline? _____

_____

_____

_____

7. Where is a Zenker's diverticulum located, and which diagnostic exam will be helpful in determining the diagnosis? _____

_____

_____

_____

8. List the symptoms of Ménière's syndrome.

_____

_____

_____

_____

9. List several reasons for nasal septal perforation.

_____

_____

_____

_____

10. What is the most frequent cause of epiglottitis?

_____

_____

_____

11. Swimmer's ear is a specific example of what more general condition? _____

_____

_____

_____

12. What are some of the causes of nasal obstruction?

_____

_____

_____

_____

13. What is the usual cause of a vocal cord nodule?

_____

_____

_____

_____

14. Define deafness. _____

_____

_____

_____

_____

15. What is the origin of a polyp? _____

_____

_____

_____

_____

■ Exercise C – Operation

1. What is the name of the procedure used to remove nasal polyps, and what special instrument may be used to perform the procedure?

_____

_____

_____

_____

2. What is the unique feature of the #12 knife blade?

_____

_____

_____

3. Are any special precautions necessary when using a carbon dioxide laser? If so, what are they?

_____

_____

_____

4. Describe the differences between rhinoplasty and septoplasty. _____

_____

_____

_____

_____

5. Which tonsils are typically removed during a tonsillectomy? _____

_____

_____

_____

_____

6. What are the reasons for reversing the operating table during ear surgery? _____

_____

_____

_____

7. Is sinus endoscopy a diagnostic or a functional procedure? Why? _____

_____

_____

_____

_____

8. An adult patient undergoing tonsillectomy with local anesthesia will be placed in what position?

_____

_____

_____

_____

9. What source of energy will be needed to operate the rotating drill? _____

_____

_____

_____

10. What is intranasal antrostomy, and what special instrument may be needed to facilitate the procedure?

_____

_____

_____

_____

11. What is the most common autologous site for securing a graft for myringoplasty?_____

_____

_____

_____

_____

12. What are the classifications for tympanoplasty, and how are they determined? _____

_____

_____

_____

_____

13. Where is the incision made to facilitate drainage of the frontal sinus? _____

_____

_____

_____

_____

14. What is the pillar dissector used for?_____

_____

_____

_____

_____

15. Describe panendoscopy, and list any special equipment that may be required. _____

_____

_____

_____

_____

_____

_____

■ Exercise D – Specific Variations

Student Name _____ Date _____

Instructor _____

Surgical Procedure – Student Case Study Report

The student will be provided with basic patient information (real or simulated) and is expected to complete the following case study.

1. Procedure name: _____

   _____

   _____

2. Definition of procedure: _____

   _____

   _____

   _____

   _____

3. What is the purpose of the procedure? _____

   _____

   _____

   _____

   _____

4. What is the expected outcome of the procedure?

   _____

   _____

   _____

   _____

5. Patient age: _____

6. Gender: _____

7. Additional pertinent patient information: _____

   _____

   _____

   _____

8. Probable preoperative diagnosis:

   _____   _____

   _____   _____

   _____   _____

   _____   _____

   _____   _____

9. How was the diagnosis determined? _____

   _____

   _____

   _____

   _____

   _____

10. Discuss the relevant anatomy. _____

    _____

    _____

    _____

    _____

    _____

    _____

11. List the general and procedure-specific equipment that will be needed for the procedure.

    _____   _____

    _____   _____

    _____   _____

    _____   _____

12. List the general and procedure-specific instruments that will be needed for the procedure.

_____ _____

_____ _____

_____ _____

_____ _____

_____ _____

_____ _____

13. List the basic and procedure-specific supplies that will be needed for the procedure.

Pack _____

Basin _____

Gloves _____

Blades _____

Drapes _____

_____

Drains _____

Dressings _____

_____

Suture—Type of Suture, Needle (if applicable), and Anticipated Tissue Usage

_____ _____

_____ _____

_____ _____

_____ _____

_____ _____

Pharmaceuticals

_____ _____

_____ _____

_____ _____

_____ _____

Miscellaneous

_____ _____

_____ _____

_____ _____

_____ _____

_____ _____

14. Operative preparation: _____

_____

_____

_____

_____

_____

_____

15. What type of anesthesia will likely be used? Why?

_____

_____

_____

_____

_____

16. List any special anesthesia equipment that may be needed. _____

_____

_____

_____

_____

_____

_____

17. Patient position during the procedure: _____

_____

_____

_____

18. What supplies will be necessary for positioning?

_____

_____

_____

_____

19. What type of shave/skin preparation will be necessary (if any)? _____

_____

_____

_____

_____

20. Define the anatomic perimeters of the prep.

_____

_____

_____

_____

_____

21. List the order in which the drapes will be applied, and describe any specific variations.

_____

_____

_____

_____

_____

_____

_____

22. List any practical considerations.

_____

_____

_____

_____

_____

_____

23. List the procedural steps, and describe the preparatory and supportive actions of the STSR during each step (use additional space if necessary).

Operative Procedure	Technical Considerations
1.	•
	•
2.	•
	•
3.	•
	•
4.	•
	•
5.	•
	•

(continues)

Operative Procedure (continued)	**Technical Considerations** (continued)
6.	•
	•
7.	•
	•
8.	•
	•
9.	•
	•
10.	•
	•

24. What is the postoperative diagnosis? _____

_____

_____

_____

_____

_____

25. Describe the immediate postoperative care.

_____

_____

_____

_____

_____

_____

26. What is the patient's long-term prognosis?

_____

_____

_____

_____

_____

27. What are the possible complications? _____

_____

_____

_____

_____

_____

_____

28. Comments or questions: _____

_____

_____

_____

_____

_____

29. What is the most valuable information you obtained from preparing this surgical procedure case study?

_____

_____

_____

_____

Case Studies

CASE STUDY 1

Stan, a 46-year-old male, is about to spend the night in the "sleep lab." After numerous complaints from his wife that his heavy snoring is keeping her awake, Stan visited his primary care physician. Following a complete physical, Stan was diagnosed with hypertension and obesity, and he was referred to an otorhinolaryngologist.

1. What tests will Stan undergo in the "sleep lab?" _____

_____

_____

_____

_____

2. What diagnosis do you think that the otorhinolaryngologist is considering? _____

_____

_____

_____

_____

3. What are Stan's conservative treatment options? _____

_____

_____

_____

_____

4. If Stan's condition eventually requires surgery, which procedure will be performed, and what structures will be removed? _____

_____

_____

_____

_____

☐ **CASE STUDY 2**

Fred, a 4-year-old male, has been placed in respite foster care because of his uncontrollable temper tantrums, which include long bouts of screaming. The foster family noticed that Fred's voice was hoarse and that it did not improve over time. He was seen by an otorhinolaryngologist, who determined that Fred has developed nodules on his vocal cords.

1. Is Fred's condition life-threatening? _____

_____

_____

_____

2. How was Fred's condition diagnosed?_____

_____

_____

_____

3. What action will be necessary to treat Fred's condition?_____

_____

_____

_____

_____

4. If surgery is required, what type of procedure will be necessary, and how will it be accomplished?

_____

_____

_____

5. If surgery is necessary, will the foster parents have the legal authority to sign his operative consent?

_____

_____

_____

_____

☐

Oral and Maxillofacial Surgery

CHAPTER 18

OBJECTIVES

After studying this chapter, the reader should be able to:

A 1. Discuss the anatomy relevant to oral and maxillofacial surgery.

P 2. Describe the pathology that prompts oral and maxillofacial surgery and the related terminology.

3. Discuss any special preoperative diagnostic procedures/tests pertaining to oral and maxillofacial surgery.

O 4. Discuss special preoperative preparation procedures related to oral and maxillofacial surgery.

5. Identify the names and uses of oral and maxillofacial instruments, supplies, and drugs.

6. Identify the names and uses of special equipment used for oral and maxillofacial surgery.

7. Discuss the intraoperative preparation of the patient undergoing an oral or maxillofacial procedure.

8. Define and give an overview of oral and maxillofacial procedures.

9. Discuss the purpose and expected outcomes of oral and maxillofacial procedures.

10. Discuss the immediate postoperative care and possible complications of oral and maxillofacial procedures.

S 11. Discuss any specific variations related to the preoperative, intraoperative, and postoperative care of the oral and maxillofacial surgical patient.

■ Select Key Terms

Define the following:

1. alveolar process _____

   _____

2. arthroscopy _____

   _____

3. calvarial _____

   _____

4. condyle _____

   _____

5. coronal flap _____

   _____

6. craniosynostosis _____

   _____

7. dentition _____

   _____

8. glenoid fossa _____

   _____

9. gnath- _____

   _____

10. labia _____

    _____

11. malar bone _____

    _____

12. malocclusion _____

    _____

13. maxillofacial _____

    _____

14. meniscus _____

    _____

15. mouth prop _____

    _____

16. orbicular _____

    _____

17. osteotomy _____

    _____

18. pan- _____

    _____

19. ramus _____

    _____

20. reduction _____

    _____

21. sagittal _____

    _____

22. symphysis _____

    _____

23. TMJ _____

    _____

■ Exercise A – Anatomy

1. Identify the bones of the anterior skull shown in Figure 18-1.

   A. _____

   B. _____

   C. _____

   D. _____

   E. _____

   F. _____

   G. _____

   H. _____

2. Identify the structures of the lateral skull shown in Figure 18-2.

   A. _____

   B. _____

   C. _____

   D. _____

   E. _____

   F. _____

   G. _____

   H. _____

   I. _____

   J. _____

   K. _____

   L. _____

   M. _____

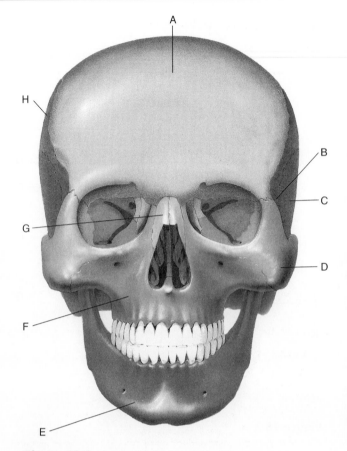

Figure 18-1

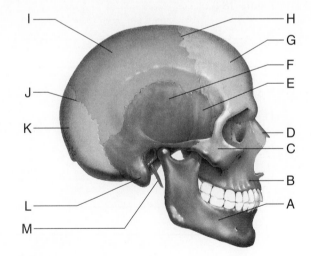

Figure 18-2

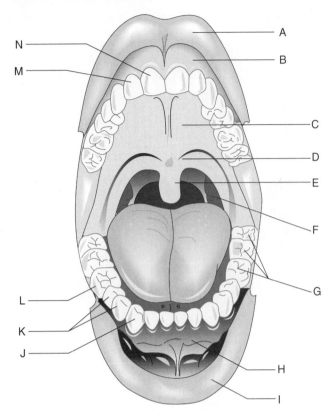

Figure 18-3

3. Identify the structures of the mouth shown in Figure 18-3.

A. _____

B. _____

C. _____

D. _____

E. _____

F. _____

G. _____

H. _____

I. _____

J. _____

K. _____

L. _____

M. _____

N. _____

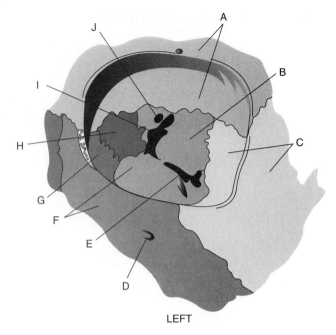

LEFT

Figure 18-4

4. Identify the structures of the orbit shown in Figure 18-4.

A. _____

B. _____

C. _____

D. _____

E. _____

F. _____

G. _____

H. _____

I. _____

J. _____

5. The anterior portion of the palate is referred to as the _____ palate.

6. What is the location and function of the soft palate?

_____

_____

_____

_____

7. The malar bone is also referred to as the _____ bone.

8. What are the inferior nasal conchae, and what is their function? _____

_____

_____

_____

_____

9. What is another name for the facial nerve? Which facial muscles are innervated by the facial nerve?

_____

_____

_____

_____

_____

10. Which four muscles control movement of the lower jaw? _____

_____

_____

_____

11. When does embryologic development of the face occur? _____

_____

_____

_____

12. Where is the orbicularis oris muscle situated? What is its function? _____

_____

_____

_____

13. Describe the components and features of the TMJ.

_____

_____

_____

_____

14. What is the ramus of the mandible?

_____

_____

_____

_____

15. What are the two main functions of the orbit?

_____

_____

_____

_____

■ Exercise B – Pathology

1. What are dental caries, and what is their cause?

_____

_____

_____

_____

2. What is meant by the term *malocclusion*? List two causes.

_____

_____

_____

_____

3. How does Paget's disease affect facial anatomy?

_____

_____

_____

_____

4. Describe a tri-malar fracture. _____

_____

_____

_____

_____

5. List the four categories of mandibular fractures.

A. _____

B. _____

C. _____

D. _____

6. What type of midfacial fracture is the most common?

_____

_____

_____

_____

7. What is laterognathism? List two causes. _____

_____

_____

A. _____

B. _____

8. What specific radiographic view is used to detect a fracture of the frontal bone? _____

_____

_____

_____

_____

9. Define cerebrospinal rhinorrhea. _____

_____

_____

_____

_____

10. List three methods for diagnosing a zygomatic fracture. _____

_____

_____

_____

_____

11. List three visual findings that could indicate the presence of a zygomatic fracture.

A. _____

B. _____

C. _____

12. Premature closure of the sutures of the skull is called _____.

13. Name and describe the four categories of tooth fractures.

A. _____

B. _____

C. _____

D. _____

14. List two advantages of three-dimensional imaging.

A. _____

B. _____

15. In addition to radiographic studies (including three-dimensional imaging), what other items may be useful to the surgeon during facial reconstruction surgery? _____

_____

_____

_____

_____

■ Exercise C – Operation

1. What is the importance of having the X-rays in the operating room prior to and during the surgical procedure? _____

   _____

   _____

   _____

   _____

2. What is accomplished by inserting a mouth prop during certain oral surgical procedures? _____

   _____

   _____

   _____

   _____

3. What is the purpose of inserting a throat pack? How is it inserted? _____

   _____

   _____

   _____

   _____

4. When is the throat pack removed? Why? _____

   _____

   _____

   _____

5. List two options for sealing an intranasal dural tear.

   A. _____

   B. _____

6. Define *autogenous*, and list two possible donor sites for autogenous bone grafts. _____

   _____

   _____

   A. _____

   B. _____

7. Why is a local anesthetic with epinephrine often injected at the operative site preoperatively when the patient is under general anesthesia? _____

   _____

   _____

   _____

   _____

8. Describe the location of a coronal incision. _____

   _____

   _____

   _____

9. List two methods for securing and positioning a soft tissue flap.

   A. _____

   B. _____

10. In what position will the patient be placed for a posterior cranial expansion? _____

   _____

   _____

   _____

11. What type of procedure is performed to treat orthognathia? _____

   _____

   _____

   _____

   _____

12. What can be done during lengthy oral procedures to prevent drying and cracking of the lips? _____

   _____

   _____

   _____

   _____

13. Why is it important to assure that all metal implants are of the same type?

_____

_____

_____

_____

14. If a bone graft is needed during a procedure in which the patient has a coronal incision, what type of bone will be considered as the first choice? Why?

_____

_____

_____

_____

15. In what situation(s) is arch bar fixation employed?

_____

_____

_____

_____

_____

_____

_____

▪ Exercise D – Specific Variations

Student Name _____ Date _____

Instructor _____

Surgical Procedure – Student Case Study Report

The student will be provided with basic patient information (real or simulated) and is expected to complete the following case study.

1. Procedure name: _____

_____

_____

2. Definition of procedure: _____

_____

_____

_____

_____

3. What is the purpose of the procedure? _____

_____

_____

_____

4. What is the expected outcome of the procedure?

_____

_____

_____

5. Patient age: _____

6. Gender: _____

7. Additional pertinent patient information: _____

_____

_____

_____

8. Probable preoperative diagnosis: _____

_____

_____

_____

9. How was the diagnosis determined? _____

_____

_____

_____

_____

10. Discuss the relevant anatomy. _____

_____

_____

_____

_____

_____

11. List the general and procedure-specific equipment that will be needed for the procedure.

_____   _____

_____   _____

_____   _____

_____   _____

_____   _____

12. List the general and procedure-specific instruments that will be needed for the procedure.

_____   _____

_____   _____

_____   _____

_____   _____

_____   _____

_____   _____

13. List the basic and procedure-specific supplies that will be needed for the procedure.

Pack _____

Basin _____

Gloves _____

Blades _____

Drapes _____

_____

Drains _____

Dressings _____

_____

Suture—Type of Suture, Needle (if applicable), and Anticipated Tissue Usage

_____   _____

_____   _____

_____   _____

_____   _____

_____   _____

Pharmaceuticals

_____   _____

_____   _____

_____   _____

_____   _____

_____   _____

Miscellaneous

_____   _____

_____   _____

_____   _____

_____   _____

_____   _____

_____   _____

14. Operative preparation: _____

_____

_____

_____

_____

_____

15. What type of anesthesia will likely be used? Why?

_____

_____

_____

_____

16. List any special anesthesia equipment that may be needed. _____

_____

_____

_____

_____

_____

17. Patient position during the procedure: _____

_____

_____

_____

18. What supplies will be necessary for positioning?

_____

_____

_____

_____

_____

19. What type of shave/skin preparation will be necessary (if any)? _____

_____

_____

_____

_____

20. Define the anatomic perimeters of the prep.

_____

_____

_____

_____

_____

21. List the order in which the drapes will be applied, and describe any specific variations.

_____

_____

_____

_____

_____

_____

22. List any practical considerations.

_____

_____

_____

_____

_____

23. List the procedural steps, and describe the preparatory and supportive actions of the STSR during each step (use additional space if necessary).

Operative Procedure	Technical Considerations
1.	•
	•
2.	•
	•
3.	•
	•
4.	•
	•
5.	•
	•

(continues)

Operative Procedure *(continued)*	Technical Considerations *(continued)*
6.	•
	•
7.	•
	•
8.	•
	•
9.	•
	•
10.	•
	•

24. What is the postoperative diagnosis? _____

_____

_____

_____

_____

25. Describe the immediate postoperative care.

_____

_____

_____

26. What is the patient's long-term prognosis?

_____

_____

_____

_____

_____

27. What are the possible complications? _____

_____

_____

_____

28. Comments or questions: _____

_____

_____

_____

_____

_____

_____

29. What is the most valuable information you obtained from preparing this surgical procedure case study?

_____

_____

_____

_____

_____

■ Case Studies

□ CASE STUDY 1

Lucricia is a 14-year-old with cerebral palsy and epilepsy. She is scheduled for dental restoration, including gingivectomy for hyperplasia of her gums, under general anesthesia.

1. What procedures may be performed during dental restoration?

   _____

   _____

   _____

   _____

2. Why is general anesthesia indicated in Lucricia's case?

   _____

   _____

   _____

   _____

3. What is the most likely reason that Lucricia suffers from hyperplasia of her gums that is severe enough to require gingivectomy?

   _____

   _____

   _____

   _____

☐ **CASE STUDY 2**

Roberto experienced a severe blow to his left cheek when he accidentally struck the corner of the wall as he was rushing through a dark hallway during the night, on his way to the bathroom. He is suffering severe pain, and it appears to him that his face no longer has a symmetrical appearance.

1. What type of injury do you suspect that Roberto has incurred? _____

_____

_____

_____

_____

2. What type of examination(s) will be performed by the maxillofacial surgeon to confirm the diagnosis?

_____

_____

_____

_____

3. How will Roberto's problem be corrected? _____

_____

_____

_____

_____

_____

☐

CHAPTER 19

Plastic and Reconstructive Surgery

OBJECTIVES

After studying this chapter, the reader should be able to:

A 1. Discuss the relevant anatomy and physiology of the skin and its underlying tissues.

P 2. Describe the pathology that prompts plastic/reconstructive surgical intervention and the related terminology.

3. Discuss any special preoperative plastic/reconstructive diagnostic procedures/tests.

O 4. Discuss any special preoperative preparation procedures related to plastic/reconstructive surgical procedures.

5. Identify the names and uses of plastic/reconstructive instruments, supplies, and drugs.

6. Identify the names and uses of special equipment related to plastic/reconstructive surgery.

7. Discuss the intraoperative preparation of the patient undergoing a plastic/reconstructive procedure.

8. Define and give an overview of the plastic/reconstructive procedure.

9. Discuss the purpose and expected outcomes of the plastic/reconstructive procedure.

10. Discuss the immediate postoperative care and possible complications of the plastic/reconstructive procedure.

S 11. Discuss any specific variations related to the preoperative, intraoperative, and postoperative care of the plastic/reconstructive patient.

■ Select Key Terms

Define the following:

1. aesthetic _____

_____

2. arthrodesis _____

_____

3. augmentation _____

_____

4. carpal tunnel _____

_____

5. cheiló- _____

_____

6. cleft _____

_____

7. dermatome _____

_____

8. elliptical _____

_____

9. ganglion cyst _____

_____

10. gynecomastia _____

_____

11. integumentary _____

_____

12. MPJ _____

_____

13. poly- _____

_____

14. radial hypoplasia _____

_____

15. replantation _____

_____

16. rhinoplasty _____

_____

17. -schisis _____

_____

18. sebum _____

_____

19. STSG _____

_____

20. syndactyly _____

_____

21. synthesis _____

_____

22. xenograft _____

_____

■ Exercise A – Anatomy

1. Identify the structures shown in Figure 19-1.

   A. _____

   B. _____

   C. _____

   D. _____

   E. _____

   F. _____

   G. _____

   H. _____

   I. _____

   J. _____

   K. _____

   L. _____

   M. _____

   N. _____

   O. _____

   P. _____

   Q. _____

2. Identify the bones of the dorsal hand shown in Figure 19-2.

   A. _____

   B. _____

   C. _____

   D. _____

   E. _____

   F. _____

   G. _____

   H. _____

   I. _____

   J. _____

   K. _____

   L. _____

   M. _____

   N. _____

   O. _____

   P. _____

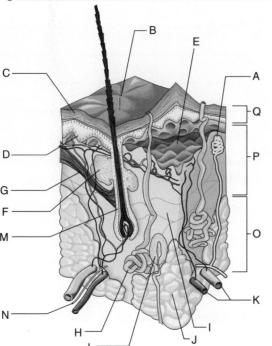

Figure 19-1

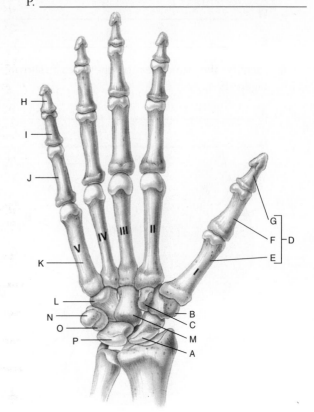

Figure 19-2

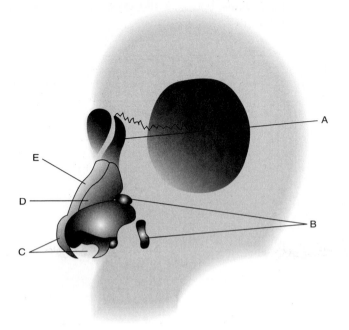

Figure 19-3

3. Identify the nasal structures shown in Figure 19-3.

A. _____

B. _____

C. _____

D. _____

E. _____

4. Identify the structures of the breast shown in Figure 19-4.

A. _____

B. _____

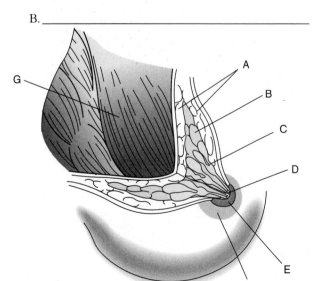

Figure 19-4

C. _____

D. _____

E. _____

F. _____

G. _____

5. Name the two major layers of the integumentary system.

A. _____

B. _____

6. List the major functions of the skin.

A. _____

B. _____

C. _____

D. _____

E. _____

F. _____

G. _____

7. Sweat glands are also known as the _____ glands.

8. Name and briefly describe the three types of sudoriferous glands.

A. _____

_____

B. _____

_____

C. _____

9. Name the structures that are contained in the anterior (palmar) compartment of the hand.

_____

_____

_____

_____

10. Development of the upper limb is complete by the _____ week in utero.

11. Name the five layers of the epidermis in sequence from outermost to innermost layer.

    A. _____

    B. _____

    C. _____

    D. _____

    E. _____

12. Name the three functions of the subcutaneous tissue layer.

    A. _____

    B. _____

    C. _____

13. Name the two divisions of the dermis, and briefly describe them.

    A. _____

    B. _____

14. Name the secretion that is produced in the sebaceous glands. What is the purpose of the secretion? _____

    _____

    _____

    _____

    _____

15. What is the function of the palate? _____

    _____

    _____

    _____

    _____

■ Exercise B – Pathology

1. Which tissue layer(s) is/are affected by a second-degree burn? _____

    _____

    _____

    _____

    _____

2. Use the Rule of Nines to determine the percentage of the body surface area affected by a third-degree burn of the chest, back, and left arm.

    _____

    _____

    _____

    _____

3. Name the bacteria that are the main causative agents of acne vulgaris.

    A. _____

    B. _____

    C. _____

4. Only 20% of cleft deformities are genetic. What is/are the cause(s) of the remaining 80%?_____

    _____

    _____

    _____

    _____

5. What is the most common type of polydactyly?

    _____

    _____

    _____

    _____

6. What is a ganglion cyst? _____

    _____

    _____

    _____

    _____

7. What causes the formation of a ganglion cyst?

    _____

    _____

    _____

    _____

8. Name three treatment options for a ganglion cyst.

   A. _____

   B. _____

   C. _____

9. What is the cause of ptosis of the eyelid?_____

   _____

   _____

   _____

   _____

10. Define neoplasm. Is a neoplasm malignant?

    _____

    _____

    _____

    _____

11. Give three examples of common malignant neoplasms of the skin.

    A. _____

    B. _____

    C. _____

12. What is the cause of cheiloschisis and palatoschisis?

    _____

    _____

    _____

    _____

13. Name two diseases of the hand that are caused by stenosing tenosynovitis.

    A. _____

    B. _____

14. List two manifestations of palmar fascia contraction (Dupuytren's disease).

    A. _____

    B. _____

15. What is the cause of rheumatoid arthritis? _____

    _____

    _____

    _____

    _____

■ Exercise C – Operation

1. Describe the difference between nasal and rhinoplasty instrumentation. _____

   _____

   _____

   _____

   _____

   _____

2. What is the purpose/function of a dermatome?

   _____

   _____

   _____

   _____

3. List two possible power sources for the oscillating-blade-type dermatome.

   A. _____

   B. _____

4. What is the purpose of a mesh graft device?

   _____

   _____

   _____

   _____

5. What is the purpose of a tacking suture? _____

   _____

   _____

   _____

   _____

6. What is the advantage of tumescent liposuction over the traditional method? _____

   _____

   _____

   _____

   _____

7. What is the common name for the umbilical template used during abdominoplasty? What is its purpose?

   _____

   _____

   _____

   _____

8. How is sterile mineral oil used during procurement of a STSG? _____

   _____

   _____

   _____

9. How is the recipient site prepared prior to placement of a STSG? Why? _____

   _____

   _____

   _____

10. Why is palatoplasty considered a clean, rather than sterile, procedure? _____

   _____

   _____

   _____

11. What anatomic area is prepped prior to draping for hand surgery? _____

   _____

   _____

   _____

12. Why is the extremity wrapped with an Esmarch bandage prior to tourniquet inflation? _____

   _____

   _____

   _____

13. Provide two indications for joint replacement in the hand.

   A. _____

   B. _____

14. Replantation of a digit begins with the attachment of which structure(s)? _____

   _____

   _____

   _____

15. List four incision options that are used to achieve augmentation mammoplasty by producing a minimal or completely hidden scar.

   A. _____

   B. _____

   C. _____

   D. _____

■ Exercise D – Specific Variations

Student Name _____ Date _____

Instructor _____

Surgical Procedure – Student Case Study Report

The student will be provided with basic patient information (real or simulated) and is expected to complete the following case study.

1. Procedure name: _____

   _____

   _____

2. Definition of procedure: _____

   _____

   _____

   _____

   _____

3. What is the purpose of the procedure? _____

   _____

   _____

   _____

   _____

4. What is the expected outcome of the procedure?

   _____

   _____

   _____

   _____

5. Patient age: _____

6. Gender: _____

7. Additional pertinent patient information: _____

   _____

   _____

   _____

8. Probable preoperative diagnosis: _____

   _____

   _____

   _____

   _____

   _____

9. How was the diagnosis determined? _____

   _____

   _____

   _____

   _____

   _____

10. Discuss the relevant anatomy. _____

    _____

    _____

    _____

    _____

    _____

11. List the general and procedure-specific equipment that will be needed for the procedure.

    _____   _____

    _____   _____

    _____   _____

    _____   _____

    _____   _____

12. List the general and procedure-specific instruments that will be needed for the procedure.

_____   _____

_____   _____

_____   _____

_____   _____

_____   _____

_____   _____

13. List the basic and procedure-specific supplies that will be needed for the procedure.

Pack _____

Basin _____

Gloves _____

Blades _____

Drapes _____

_____

Drains _____

Dressings _____

_____

Suture—Type of Suture, Needle (if applicable), and Anticipated Tissue Usage

_____   _____

_____   _____

_____   _____

_____   _____

_____   _____

Pharmaceuticals

_____   _____

_____   _____

_____   _____

_____   _____

_____   _____

Miscellaneous

_____   _____

_____   _____

_____   _____

_____   _____

_____   _____

_____   _____

14. Operative preparation: _____

_____

_____

_____

_____

_____

15. What type of anesthesia will likely be used? Why?

_____

_____

_____

_____

_____

16. List any special anesthesia equipment that may be needed. _____

_____

_____

_____

_____

_____

17. Patient position during the procedure: _____

_____

_____

_____

18. What supplies will be necessary for positioning?

    _____

    _____

    _____

    _____

    _____

19. What type of shave/skin preparation will be necessary (if any)? _____

    _____

    _____

    _____

    _____

20. Define the anatomic perimeters of the prep.

    _____

    _____

    _____

    _____

    _____

21. List the order in which the drapes will be applied, and describe any specific variations.

    _____

    _____

    _____

    _____

    _____

    _____

    _____

    _____

22. List any practical considerations.

    _____

    _____

    _____

    _____

    _____

    _____

23. List the procedural steps, and describe the preparatory and supportive actions of the STSR during each step (use additional space if necessary).

Operative Procedure	Technical Considerations
1.	•
	•
2.	•
	•
3.	•
	•
4.	•
	•
5.	•
	•

Operative Procedure *(continued)*	Technical Considerations *(continued)*
6.	•
	•
7.	•
	•
8.	•
	•
9.	•
	•
10.	•
	•

24. What is the postoperative diagnosis? _____

_____

_____

_____

_____

25. Describe the immediate postoperative care.

_____

_____

_____

_____

_____

26. What is the patient's long-term prognosis?

_____

_____

_____

_____

_____

27. What are the possible complications? _____

_____

_____

_____

_____

_____

_____

28. Comments or questions: _____

_____

_____

_____

_____

_____

_____

29. What is the most valuable information you obtained from preparing this surgical procedure case study?

_____

_____

_____

_____

■ Case Studies

□ CASE STUDY 1

Three-year-old Bobby accidentally pulled on the tablecloth, causing his mother's scalding coffee to spill on his left neck, shoulder, and chest. It has been determined that Bobby has suffered second- and third-degree burns over 9% of his body. The accident occurred three weeks ago, and Bobby is now scheduled for a STSG.

1. How was the extent of Bobby's injury determined? _____

    _____

    _____

    _____

    _____

2. What was the biggest risk that Bobby faced with the third-degree burns? _____

    _____

    _____

    _____

    _____

3. What is "STSG," and what special instrument will be required to obtain the graft?_____

    _____

    _____

    _____

    _____

4. From which anatomic site is the graft most likely to be procured? _____

    _____

    _____

    _____

    _____

☐ CASE STUDY 2

Sven is a 62-year-old dairy farmer. He has been diagnosed with Dupuytren's disease. The disease has progressed to the point where Sven is unable to use his right hand effectively to connect the milking machine to his cows. He has put off surgery as long as possible, but now the inevitable has arrived.

1. What is Dupuytren's disease?

   _____

   _____

   _____

   _____

2. Is the condition painful?

   _____

   _____

   _____

   _____

3. What procedure will be necessary to treat Sven's condition?

   _____

   _____

   _____

   _____

4. Can Sven expect to regain full function and normal appearance?

   _____

   _____

   _____

   _____

   ☐

CHAPTER
20

Genitourinary Surgery

OBJECTIVES

After studying this chapter, the reader should be able to:

A   1. Discuss the relevant anatomy of the genitourinary system.

P   2. Describe the pathology that prompts genitourinary system surgical intervention and the related terminology.

     3. Discuss any special preoperative genitourinary diagnostic procedures/tests.

O   4. Discuss any special preoperative genitourinary preparation procedures.

     5. Identify the names and uses of genitourinary instruments, supplies, and drugs.

     6. Identify the names and uses of special genitourinary equipment.

     7. Discuss the intraoperative preparation of the patient undergoing the genitourinary procedure.

     8. Define and give an overview of the genitourinary procedure.

     9. Discuss the purpose and expected outcomes of the genitourinary procedure.

   10. Discuss the immediate postoperative care and possible complications of the genitourinary procedure.

S   11. Discuss any specific variations related to the preoperative, intraoperative, and postoperative care of the genitourinary patient.

Select Key Terms

Define the following:

1. ACTH _____

_____

2. afferent _____

_____

3. calculi _____

_____

4. conduit _____

_____

5. cortex _____

_____

6. ESWL _____

_____

7. focal point _____

_____

8. Gerota's fascia _____

_____

9. Gibson incision _____

_____

10. hilum _____

_____

11. hirsutism _____

_____

12. hypertrophy _____

_____

13. hypospadias _____

_____

14. incontinence _____

_____

15. intravenous urogram (IVU) _____

_____

16. medulla _____

_____

17. prepuce _____

_____

18. retroperitoneal _____

_____

19. stoma _____

_____

20. suprarenal glands _____

_____

21. torsion _____

_____

22. TURP _____

_____

23. UTI _____

_____

24. vesical trigone _____

_____

■ **Exercise A – Anatomy**

1. Identify the structures shown in Figure 20-1.

A. _____

B. _____

C. _____

D. _____

E. _____

F. _____

G. _____

H. _____

I. _____

J. _____

K. _____

L. _____

M. _____

N. _____

O. _____

P. _____

Q. _____

R. _____

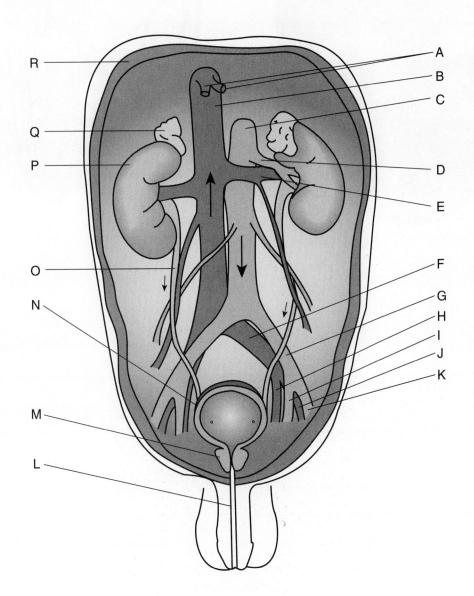

Figure 20-1

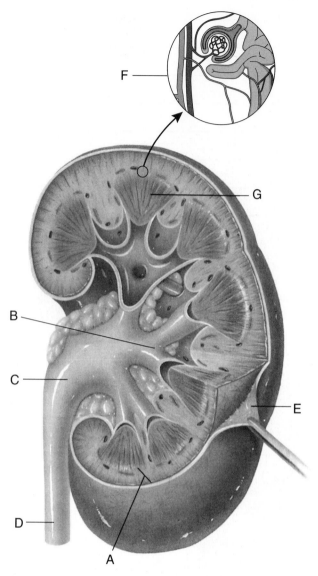

Figure 20-2

Figure 20-3

2. Identify the structures shown in Figure 20-2.

A. _____

B. _____

C. _____

D. _____

E. _____

F. _____

G. _____

3. Identify the structures shown in Figure 20-3.

A. _____

B. _____

C. _____

D. _____

E. _____

F. _____

G. _____

H. _____

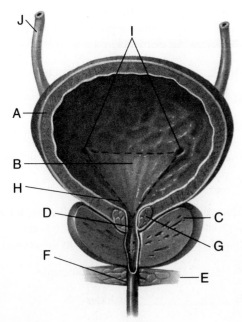

Figure 20-4

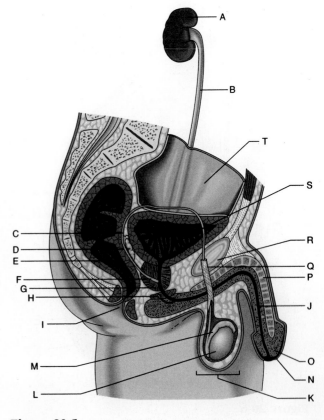

Figure 20-5

4. Identify the structures shown in Figure 20-4.

A. _____

B. _____

C. _____

D. _____

E. _____

F. _____

G. _____

H. _____

I. _____

J. _____

5. Identify the structures shown in Figure 20-5.

A. _____

B. _____

C. _____

D. _____

E. _____

F. _____

G. _____

H. _____

I. _____

J. _____

K. _____

L. _____

M. _____

N. _____

O. _____

P. _____

Q. _____

R. _____

S. _____

T. _____

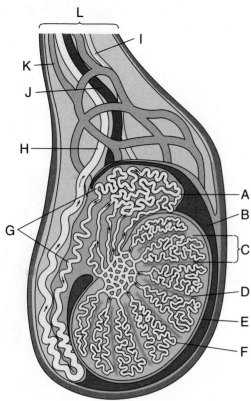

L

I

K

J

H

A
B
C
D
E
F

G

Figure 20-6

6. Identify the structures shown in Figure 20-6.

A. _____

B. _____

C. _____

D. _____

E. _____

F. _____

G. _____

H. _____

I. _____

J. _____

K. _____

L. _____

7. Trace the pathway that sperm cells follow through the ducts of the male reproductive system by placing the following elements in the correct order.

A. _____ Ductus deferens

B. _____ Ejaculatory duct

C. _____ Epididymis

D. _____ Seminiferous tubules (testis)

E. _____ Urethra

8. Trace the pathway of fluid from the time it leaves the circulatory system until it leaves the body as urine by placing the following elements in the correct order.

A. _____ Afferent arteriole

B. _____ Bladder

C. _____ Bowman's capsule

D. _____ Calyx

E. _____ Collecting tubule

F. _____ Distal convoluted tubule

G. _____ Glomerulus

H. _____ Loop of Henle

I. _____ Proximal convoluted tubule

J. _____ Renal artery

K. _____ Renal pelvis

L. _____ Ureter

M. _____ Urethra

9. Name the two portions of the adrenal gland and the function of each.

A. _____

_____

B. _____

_____

10. Describe the location of the kidneys. _____

_____

_____

_____

_____

11. By what mechanism(s) is/are urine conducted from the kidney to the bladder? _____

12. What are the anatomic boundaries of the trigone of the bladder? _____

13. Name the three cavernous structures of the penis.

    A. _____

    B. _____

    C. _____

14. What is the function of the detrusor muscle?

15. What are the functional units of the kidney, and approximately how many are located within each kidney? _____

■ Exercise B – Pathology

1. List two possible causes for Cushing's syndrome and the possible treatments for each.

    A. _____

    B. _____

2. What is pheochromocytoma? List the classic symptoms. _____

3. List the four basic chemical types of urinary calculi and their causes.

    A. _____

    B. _____

    C. _____

    D. _____

4. What is the recurrence rate of urinary calculi? What can be done to reduce the possibility of recurrence?

5. Why is family history an important factor in the diagnosis of PKD? _____

6. Name two conditions of the kidney that often lead to ESRD.

    A. _____

    B. _____

7. What are the two treatment options for a patient with ESRD?

    A. _____

    B. _____

8. What age group is most commonly affected by BPH? Why? _____

_____

_____

_____

_____

9. Is it possible for hypospadias to occur in a female patient? _____

_____

_____

_____

_____

10. List two complications that may occur if cryptorchidism is undiagnosed or untreated.

A. _____

B. _____

11. What is the normal blood level of PSA? Does an elevated PSA indicate the presence of a malignant process? _____

_____

_____

_____

12. An IVU has been unsuccessful in demonstrating a ureteral obstruction. What diagnostic exam may be recommended as the next step? _____

_____

_____

_____

13. Table 20-6 in the textbook lists the abnormal constituents of urine. If a patient exhibits an increase in leukocytes, what condition(s) could this indicate?

_____

_____

_____

14. What condition is the MIBG nuclear medicine study designed to detect? _____

_____

_____

_____

_____

15. What is KUB? What information may be provided during this type of exam? _____

_____

_____

_____

_____

■ Exercise C – Operation

1. A retrograde urogram is considered a diagnostic radiographic procedure. Why is it often performed in the operating room rather than the radiology department? _____

_____

_____

_____

_____

2. List at least three features of the Cysto Room that may not be found in the general OR. _____

_____

_____

_____

_____

_____

_____

3. What is the function of a deflecting mechanism?

_____

_____

_____

4. What is the purpose of an O'Connor shield?

_____

_____

_____

_____

_____

5. What specific structure is the Gibson incision designed to access? _____

_____

_____

_____

_____

6. In which position is the patient placed when use of a flank incision is anticipated? _____

_____

_____

_____

_____

7. List the three flank incision options and give a brief description of the location of each.

A. _____

_____

B. _____

_____

C. _____

_____

8. What is the purpose of renal cooling?

_____

_____

_____

_____

_____

_____

9. Why is it important for the STSR to have a chest tube, insertion supplies, and a water-seal drainage system readily available during a nephrectomy?

_____

_____

_____

_____

_____

_____

_____

10. List the three sources from which kidneys are obtained for transplant.

A. _____

B. _____

C. _____

11. What is the purpose of suprapubic cystostomy?

_____

_____

_____

_____

_____

12. Will the surgical technologist be scrubbed in for cystoscopy? What is the main function of the surgical technologist during cystoscopy? _____

_____

_____

_____

_____

13. List four procedures that may be performed transurethrally.

A. _____

B. _____

C. _____

D. _____

14. Why is it necessary for the assistant to change the gloves (and possibly the gown) during MMK?

_____

_____

_____

_____

15. What is the purpose of repeatedly introducing the cystoscope during a Stamey procedure?_____

_____

_____

_____

_____

■ Exercise D – Specific Variations

Student Name _____ Date _____

Instructor _____

The student will be provided with basic patient information (real or simulated) and is expected to complete the following case study.

1. Procedure name: _____

   _____

   _____

2. Definition of procedure: _____

   _____

   _____

   _____

3. What is the purpose of the procedure? _____

   _____

   _____

   _____

4. What is the expected outcome of the procedure?

   _____

   _____

   _____

5. Patient age: _____

6. Gender: _____

7. Additional pertinent patient information: _____

   _____

   _____

   _____

8. Probable preoperative diagnosis: _____

   _____

   _____

   _____

   _____

9. How was the diagnosis determined? _____

   _____

   _____

   _____

   _____

10. Discuss the relevant anatomy. _____

    _____

    _____

    _____

11. List the general and procedure-specific equipment that will be needed for the procedure.

    _____   _____

    _____   _____

    _____   _____

    _____   _____

    _____   _____

    _____   _____

12. List the general and procedure-specific instruments that will be needed for the procedure.

_____   _____

_____   _____

_____   _____

_____   _____

_____   _____

_____   _____

13. List the basic and procedure-specific supplies that will be needed for the procedure.

Pack _____

Basin _____

Gloves _____

Blades _____

Drapes _____

_____

Drains _____

Dressings _____

_____

Suture—Type of Suture, Needle (if applicable), and Anticipated Tissue Usage

_____   _____

_____   _____

_____   _____

_____   _____

Pharmaceuticals

_____   _____

_____   _____

_____   _____

_____   _____

Miscellaneous

_____   _____

_____   _____

_____   _____

_____   _____

_____   _____

14. Operative preparation: _____

_____

_____

_____

_____

_____

_____

15. What type of anesthesia will likely be used? Why?

_____

_____

_____

_____

16. List any special anesthesia equipment that may be needed.

_____

_____

_____

_____

17. Patient position during the procedure: _____

_____

_____

_____

18. What supplies will be necessary for positioning?

_____

_____

_____

_____

19. What type of shave/skin preparation will be necessary (if any)? _____

_____

_____

_____

20. Define the anatomic perimeters of the prep.

_____

_____

_____

_____

21. List the order in which the drapes will be applied, and describe any specific variations.

_____

_____

_____

_____

_____

_____

_____

22. List any practical considerations.

_____

_____

_____

_____

_____

_____

23. List the procedural steps, and describe the preparatory and supportive actions of the STSR during each step (use additional space if necessary).

Operative Procedure	Technical Considerations
1.	•
	•
2.	•
	•
3.	•
	•
4.	•
	•
5.	•
	•

(continues)

Operative Procedure *(continued)*	Technical Considerations *(continued)*
6.	•
	•
7.	•
	•
8.	•
	•
9.	•
	•
10.	•
	•

24. What is the postoperative diagnosis? _____

_____

_____

_____

_____

_____

25. Describe the immediate postoperative care.

_____

_____

_____

_____

_____

_____

26. What is the patient's long-term prognosis?

_____

_____

_____

_____

_____

_____

27. What are the possible complications? _____

_____

_____

_____

_____

_____

_____

_____

28. Comments or questions: _____

_____

_____

_____

_____

_____

_____

29. What is the most valuable information you obtained from preparing this surgical procedure case study?

_____

_____

_____

_____

_____

■ **Case Studies**

□ **CASE STUDY 1**

Patricia has been experiencing several seemingly unrelated symptoms that include weight loss, headache, "heartburn," sweating, trembling, rapid heart rate, heat intolerance, and a feeling of anxiousness. Patricia's daughter finally convinced her to see her primary care physician, who has determined that Patricia has a tumor of the adrenal medulla.

1. What diagnostic studies are needed to confirm the diagnosis?

   _____

   _____

   _____

   _____

2. What is the name of Patricia's tumor, and how serious is it? Why?

   _____

   _____

   _____

   _____

3. What is the necessary treatment for Patricia's condition? What type of procedure will most likely be performed?

   _____

   _____

   _____

   _____

□

☐ CASE STUDY 2

Six-year-old Belinda has been suffering from chronic urinary tract infections. The appearance of blood in her urine led to further testing that produced a diagnosis of PKD. Belinda's condition has nearly destroyed both kidneys. Belinda, her parents, and her twin sister, Melinda, are all extremely concerned about Belinda's future.

1. What does PKD mean, and from what type of PKD does Belinda suffer? _____

   _____

   _____

   _____

   _____

2. What does the term *parenchyma* mean? What are the parenchymatous organs? _____

   _____

   _____

   _____

   _____

3. Was invasive testing necessary to determine Belinda's diagnosis? _____

   _____

   _____

   _____

   _____

4. What course is the disease expected to follow? _____

   _____

   _____

   _____

   _____

5. What will be the most likely outcome for Belinda? _____

   _____

   _____

   _____

   _____

☐

CHAPTER
21

Orthopedic Surgery

OBJECTIVES

After studying this chapter, the reader should be able to:

A 1. Discuss the relevant anatomy and physiology of the musculoskeletal system.

P 2. Describe the pathology of the musculoskeletal system that prompts surgical intervention and the related terminology.

3. Discuss any special preoperative orthopedic diagnostic procedures/tests.

O 4. Discuss any special preoperative preparation related to orthopedic procedures.

5. Identify the names and uses of orthopedic instruments, supplies, and drugs.

6. Identify the names and uses of special equipment related to orthopedic procedures.

7. Discuss the intraoperative preparation of the patient undergoing an orthopedic procedure.

8. Define and give an overview of the orthopedic procedure.

9. Discuss the purpose and expected outcomes of the orthopedic procedure.

10. Discuss the immediate postoperative care and possible complications of the orthopedic procedure.

S 11. Discuss any specific variations related to the preoperative, intraoperative, and postoperative care of the orthopedic patient.

■ Key Terms

Define the following:

1. abduction _____

   _____

2. AC joint _____

   _____

3. adduction _____

   _____

4. amphiarthrosis _____

   _____

5. cancellous bone _____

   _____

6. cartilage _____

   _____

7. comminuted _____

   _____

8. compound fracture _____

   _____

9. cortical bone _____

   _____

10. diarthrosis _____

    _____

11. epiphysis _____

    _____

12. flexion _____

    _____

13. ligament _____

    _____

14. marrow _____

    _____

15. osteogenesis _____

    _____

16. pedicle _____

    _____

17. proximal _____

    _____

18. shoulder joint _____

    _____

19. splint _____

    _____

20. valgus _____

    _____

■ Exercise A – Anatomy

1. Identify the skeletal bones shown in Figure 21-1.

A. _____

B. _____

C. _____

D. _____

E. _____

F. _____

G. _____

H. _____

I. _____

J. _____

K. _____

L. _____

M. _____

N. _____

O. _____

P. _____

Q. _____

R. _____

S. _____

T. _____

U. _____

V. _____

W. _____

X. _____

Y. _____

Z. _____

AA. _____

BB. _____

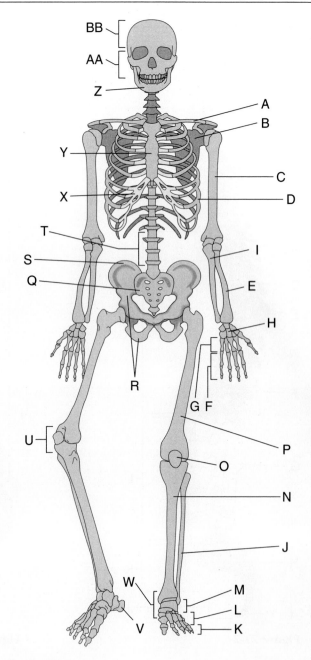

Figure 21-1

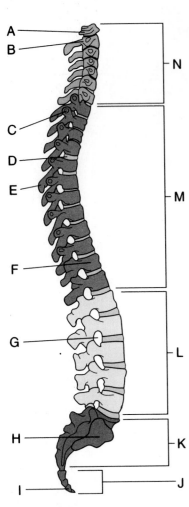

Figure 21-2

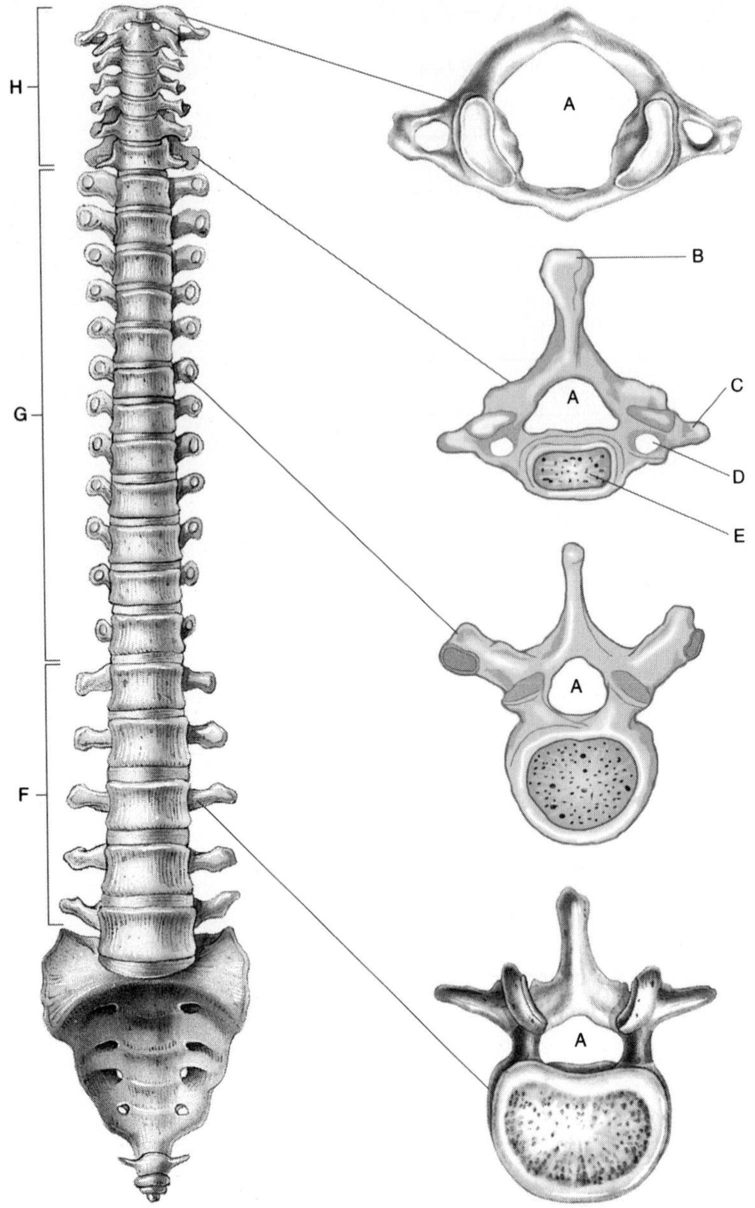

Figure 21-3

2. Identify the structures of the vertebral column shown in Figure 21-2.

A. _____

B. _____

C. _____

D. _____

E. _____

F. _____

G. _____

H. _____

I. _____

J. _____

K. _____

L. _____

M. _____

N. _____

3. Identify the vertebral structures shown in Figure 21-3.

A._____

B._____

C._____

D._____

E._____

F._____

G._____

H._____

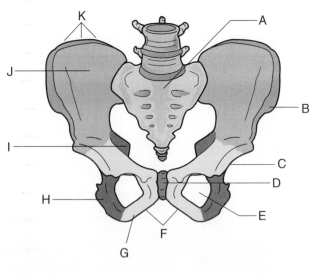

Figure 21-5

4. Identify the structures shown in Figure 21-4.

A._____

B._____

C._____

D._____

E._____

F._____

C._____

D._____

E._____

F._____

G._____

H._____

5. Identify the bones of the pelvic girdle shown in Figure 21-5.

A._____

B._____

I._____

J._____

K._____

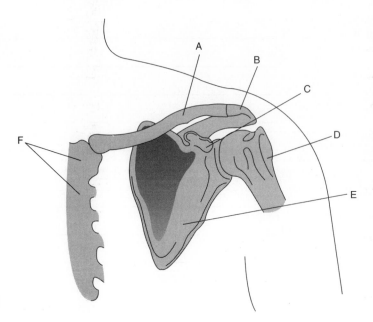

Figure 21-4

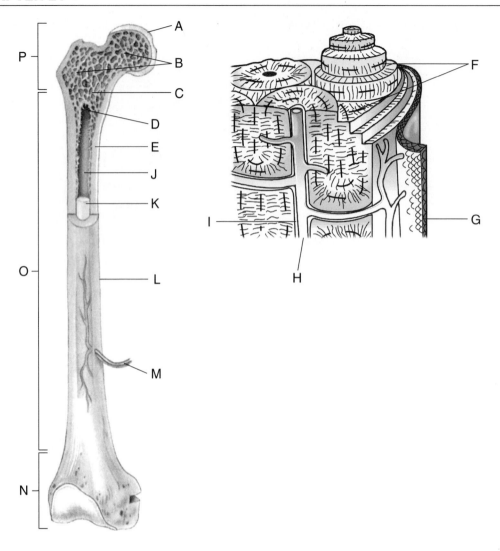

Figure 21-6

6. Identify the elements of a long bone as shown in Figure 21-6.

A. _____

B. _____

C. _____

D. _____

E. _____

F. _____

G. _____

H. _____

I. _____

J. _____

K. _____

L. _____

M. _____

N. _____

O. _____

P. _____

7. List the five functions of the skeletal system.

    A. _____

    B. _____

    C. _____

    D. _____

    E. _____

8. List four factors that affect bone growth.

    A. _____

    B. _____

    C. _____

    D. _____

9. Define the term *sesamoid*, and give two examples of sesamoid bones. _____

    _____

    _____

    A. _____

    B. _____

10. What are the two main divisions of the skeleton? Briefly describe each division.

    A. _____

    _____

    B. _____

    _____

11. List the eight bones of the cranium.

    A. _____

    B. _____

    C. _____

    D. _____

    E. _____

    F. _____

    G. _____

    H. _____

12. Name the three bones that comprise the knee joint.

    A. _____

    B. _____

    C. _____

13. Describe the function of a gliding joint, and provide an example of a gliding joint. _____

    _____

    _____

    _____

    _____

    _____

14. Define circumduction, and give an example of a joint that is capable of circumduction. _____

    _____

    _____

    _____

    _____

    _____

15. In addition to calcium, name four other minerals that are stored within bone.

    A. _____

    B. _____

    C. _____

    D. _____

■ Exercise B – Pathology

1. What is ankylosis, and what is its cause? _____

    _____

    _____

    _____

    _____

    _____

2. How does vitamin D help to prevent osteomalacia?

   _____

   _____

   _____

   _____

3. Describe a greenstick fracture. _____

   _____

   _____

   _____

   _____

4. Does a patient suffering from subluxation have a fracture? Explain your answer. _____

   _____

   _____

   _____

   _____

5. Describe nonunion, and provide two reasons why nonunion may occur. _____

   _____

   _____

   _____

   _____

6. What is the cause of compartmental syndrome? How is compartmental syndrome manifested?

   _____

   _____

   _____

   _____

7. Why is the Lachman and Drawer examination performed? _____

   _____

   _____

   _____

   _____

8. What is the main complication of osteoporosis?

   _____

   _____

   _____

   _____

9. What bone is affected by a Colles' fracture?

   _____

   _____

   _____

   _____

10. A tumor of the cartilage is called a(n) _____

11. What is the most common type of meniscal tear? Describe the defect. _____

    _____

    _____

    _____

    _____

    _____

12. _____ is an inflammation of the bone and bone marrow.

13. An elevated erythrocyte sedimentation rate (ESR) is an indicator of what type of condition?

    _____

    _____

    _____

14. What muscles comprise the rotator cuff? How will a tear of one or more of these muscles or their tendinous attachments affect the shoulder?

    _____

    _____

    _____

    _____

    _____

15. An arthrogram is an X-ray of what specific structure(s)? _____

_____

_____

_____

_____

■ Exercise C – Operation

1. What is meant by the term *exsanguination?* How does this apply to extremity surgery with the use of a tourniquet? _____

_____

_____

_____

_____

_____

2. What is the maximum recommended time that tourniquet pressure may be applied to an upper extremity? Why? _____

_____

_____

_____

_____

_____

3. What are two advantages to postoperative use of the CPM machine?

   A. _____

   B. _____

4. What precautions must be taken when the use of a C-Arm is expected? _____

_____

_____

_____

_____

_____

5. Describe the direction of the blade motion of a reciprocating saw. _____

_____

_____

_____

_____

_____

6. What is bone wax, and how is it used? _____

_____

_____

_____

_____

7. List two situations in which a bone graft may be required.

   A. _____

   B. _____

8. What is the reason for application of irrigation fluid to the wound when sawing or drilling bone?

_____

_____

_____

_____

9. When using MMA, what is the importance of using a closed mixing system?_____

_____

_____

_____

_____

10. What information must be documented following prosthesis insertion?

   A. _____

   B. _____

   C. _____

   D._____

11. List two reasons why arthroscopy may be performed.

    A. _____

    B. _____

12. What is a reamer used to accomplish?

    _____

    _____

    _____

    _____

13. What are the three main advantages of maintaining laminar airflow in the OR during a surgical procedure?

    A. _____

    B. _____

    C. _____

14. Following closed reduction, what method of immobilization is commonly employed? _____

    _____

    _____

    _____

    _____

    _____

15. List the three types of traction.

    A. _____

    B. _____

    C. _____

■ Exercise D – Specific Variations

Student Name _____ Date _____

Instructor _____

The student will be provided with basic patient information (real or simulated) and is expected to complete the following case study.

1. Procedure name: _____

   _____

   _____

2. Definition of procedure: _____

   _____

   _____

   _____

   _____

3. What is the purpose of the procedure? _____

   _____

   _____

   _____

   _____

4. What is the expected outcome of the procedure?

   _____

   _____

   _____

   _____

5. Patient age: _____

6. Gender: _____

7. Additional pertinent patient information: _____

   _____

   _____

   _____

8. Probable preoperative diagnosis: _____

   _____

   _____

   _____

   _____

   _____

9. How was the diagnosis determined? _____

   _____

   _____

   _____

   _____

10. Discuss the relevant anatomy. _____

    _____

    _____

    _____

    _____

    _____

11. List the general and procedure-specific equipment that will be needed for the procedure.

    _____   _____

    _____   _____

    _____   _____

    _____   _____

    _____   _____

12. List the general and procedure-specific instruments that will be needed for the procedure.

_____   _____

_____   _____

_____   _____

_____   _____

_____   _____

_____   _____

13. List the basic and procedure-specific supplies that will be needed for the procedure.

Pack _____

Basin _____

Gloves _____

Blades _____

Drapes _____

_____

Drains _____

Dressings _____

_____

Suture—Type of Suture, Needle (if applicable), and Anticipated Tissue Usage

_____   _____

_____   _____

_____   _____

_____   _____

_____   _____

_____   _____

_____   _____

Pharmaceuticals

_____   _____

_____   _____

_____   _____

_____   _____

_____   _____

Miscellaneous

_____   _____

_____   _____

_____   _____

_____   _____

_____   _____

_____   _____

14. Operative preparation: _____

_____

_____

_____

_____

_____

15. What type of anesthesia will likely be used? Why?

_____

_____

_____

_____

16. List any special anesthesia equipment that may be needed. _____

_____

_____

_____

_____

_____

17. Patient position during the procedure: _____

_____

_____

_____

18. What supplies will be necessary for positioning?

_____

_____

_____

_____

_____

19. What type of shave/skin preparation will be necessary (if any)?_____

_____

_____

_____

_____

20. Define the anatomic perimeters of the prep.

_____

_____

_____

_____

_____

21. List the order in which the drapes will be applied, and describe any specific variations.

_____

_____

_____

_____

_____

22. List any practical considerations.

_____

_____

_____

_____

_____

23. List the procedural steps, and describe the preparatory and supportive actions of the STSR during each step (use additional space if necessary).

Operative Procedure	Technical Considerations
1.	•
	•
2.	•
	•
3.	•
	•
4.	•
	•
5.	•
	•

(continues)

Operative Procedure (continued)	**Technical Considerations** (continued)
6.	•
	•
7.	•
	•
8.	•
	•
9.	•
	•
10.	•
	•

24. What is the postoperative diagnosis? _____

_____

_____

_____

_____

25. Describe the immediate postoperative care.

_____

_____

_____

_____

26. What is the patient's long-term prognosis?

_____

_____

_____

_____

_____

27. What are the possible complications? _____

_____

_____

_____

_____

_____

_____

28. Comments or questions: _____

_____

_____

_____

_____

_____

_____

29. What is the most valuable information you obtained from preparing this surgical procedure case study?

_____

_____

_____

_____

■ Case Studies

□ CASE STUDY 1

Ellenor is a 65-year-old female who was admitted to the hospital for a total hip arthroplasty.

1. Describe a routine draping procedure for this case. _____

   _____

   _____

   _____

   _____

2. What kind of incision is used? _____

   _____

   _____

   _____

   _____

3. After the femoral osteotomy guide is placed over the lateral femur and neck, what should the STSR plan to do next? _____

   _____

   _____

   _____

   _____

4. Will the incision be drained?_____

   _____

   _____

   _____

   _____

5. Describe the immediate postoperative care the patient will receive._____

   _____

   _____

   _____

   _____

☐ CASE STUDY 2

Leroy was admitted to the emergency department with a fracture of the left tibia and fibula. The fracture was reduced, the leg placed in a cast, and Leroy was sent home.

1. Why are casts placed on limbs with reduced fractures? _____
   _____
   _____
   _____
   _____

2. What is the meaning of the term *distraction*? What complications can be caused by distraction? _____
   _____
   _____
   _____
   _____

3. What is the most important factor in bone healing? _____
   _____
   _____
   _____
   _____

4. To what does the term *delayed union* refer? _____
   _____
   _____
   _____
   _____

   ☐

CHAPTER 22

Cardiothoracic Surgery

OBJECTIVES

After studying this chapter, the reader should be able to:

A 1. Discuss the relevant anatomy of the cardiovascular and respiratory systems.

P 2. Describe the pathology that prompts cardiac or thoracic surgical intervention and the related terminology.

3. Discuss any special preoperative diagnostic procedures/tests for the patient undergoing cardiac or thoracic surgery.

O 4. Discuss any special preoperative preparation procedures.

5. Identify the names and uses of cardiovascular and thoracic instruments, supplies, and drugs.

6. Identify the names and uses of special equipment for the cardiac or thoracic procedure.

7. Discuss the intraoperative preparation of the patient undergoing a cardiac or thoracic procedure.

8. Define and give an overview of the cardiac or thoracic procedure.

9. Discuss the purpose and expected outcomes of the cardiac or thoracic procedure.

10. Discuss the immediate postoperative care and possible complications of the cardiac or thoracic procedure.

S 11. Discuss any specific variations related to the preoperative, intraoperative, and postoperative care of the patient undergoing a cardiac or thoracic procedure.

■ **Select Key Terms**

Define the following:

1. alveoli _____

_____

2. aneurysm _____

_____

3. arrhythmia _____

_____

4. atria _____

_____

5. bradycardia _____

_____

6. cardiac cycle _____

_____

7. ductus arteriosus _____

_____

8. hyaline cartilage _____

_____

9. infarction _____

_____

10. infiltrate _____

_____

11. mediastinum _____

12. myocardium _____

_____

13. oxygenated _____

_____

14. pericardium _____

_____

15. pleura _____

_____

16. prolapse _____

_____

17. PVC _____

_____

18. regurgitation _____

_____

19. stent _____

_____

20. systole _____

_____

21. tachycardia _____

_____

22. tamponade _____

_____

23. ventricles _____

_____

■ Exercise A – Anatomy

1. Identify the structures shown in Figure 22-1.

   A. _____

   B. _____

   C. _____

   D. _____

   E. _____

2. Identify the structures shown in Figure 22-2.

   A. _____

   B. _____

   C. _____

   D. _____

   E. _____

   F. _____

   G. _____

   H. _____

   I. _____

   J. _____

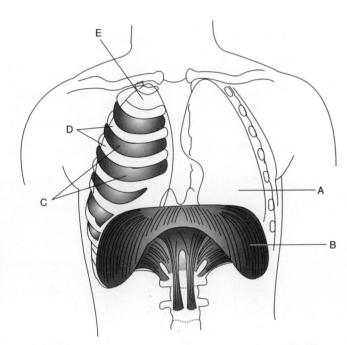

Figure 22-1

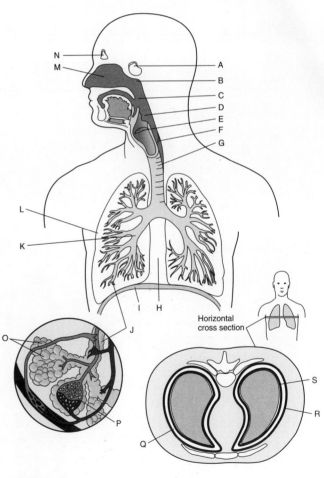

Figure 22-2

K. _____   H. _____

L. _____   I. _____

M. _____   J. _____

N. _____   K. _____

O. _____   L. _____

P. _____   M. _____

Q. _____   N. _____

R. _____   O. _____

S. _____   P. _____

3. Identify the structures shown in Figure 22-3.   Q. _____

A. _____   R. _____

B. _____   S. _____

C. _____   T. _____

D. _____   U. _____

E. _____   V. _____

F. _____   W. _____

G. _____   X. _____

Y. _____

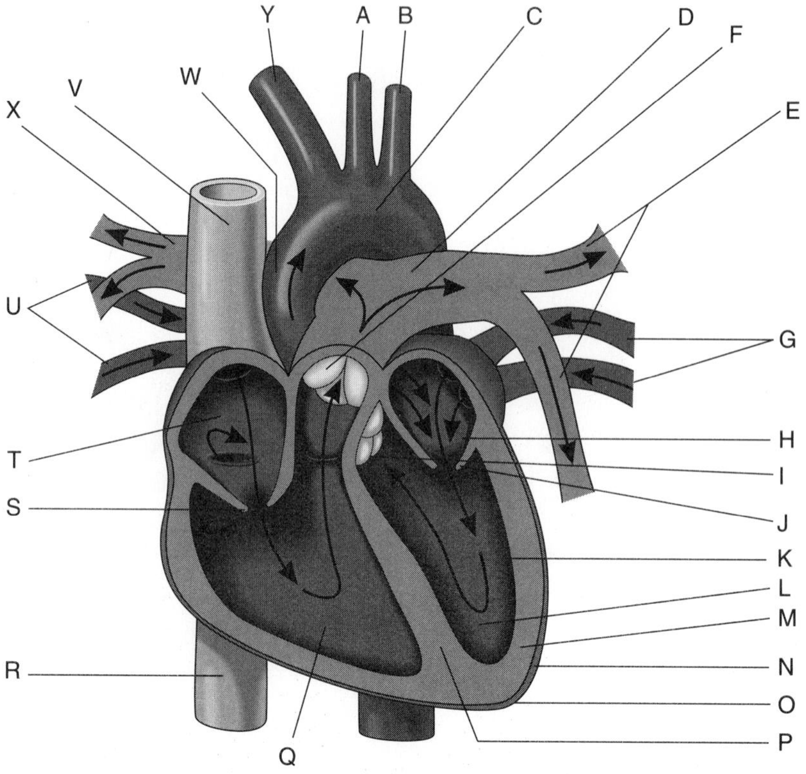

Figure 22-3

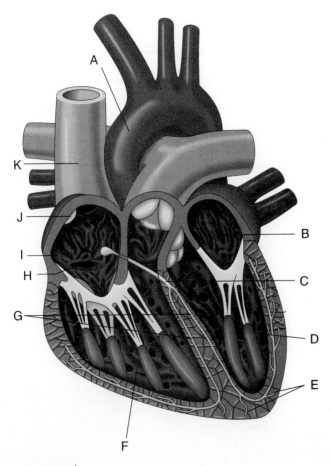

Figure 22-4

4. Identify the structures shown in Figure 22-4.

A. _____

B. _____

C. _____

D. _____

E. _____

F. _____

G. _____

H. _____

I. _____

J. _____

K. _____

5. Identify the cardiac valves shown in Figure 22-5.

A. _____

B. _____

C. _____

6. Identify the structures shown in Figure 22-6.

A. _____

B. _____

C. _____

D. _____

E. _____

F. _____

G. _____

H. _____

I. _____

J. _____

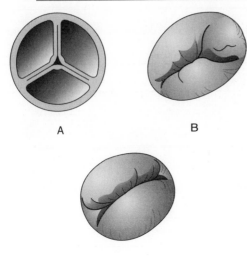

Figure 22-5

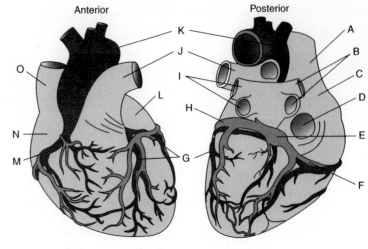

Figure 22-6

K._____

L._____

M._____

N._____

O._____

7. List the following events in the proper chronological sequence to complete the cardiac cycle.

 A. _____ Atria contract

 B. _____ AV node stimulated

 C. _____ Impulse moves through right and left bundle branches

 D. _____ Impulse transmitted to bundle of His

 E. _____ Impulse travels via internodal atrial pathways

 F. _____ Purkinje fibers stimulated

 G. _____ SA node generates initial impulse

 H. _____ Ventricles contract

8. Trace the flow of blood from the time it leaves the venae cavae to the time it enters the aorta by placing the following elements in the correct order.

 A. _____ Aorta

 B. _____ Aortic (semilunar) valve

 C. _____ Bicuspid (mitral) valve

 D. _____ Left atrium

 E. _____ Left ventricle

 F. _____ Lungs

 G. _____ Pulmonary arteries

 H. _____ Pulmonary valve

 I. _____ Pulmonary veins

 J. _____ Right atrium

 K. _____ Right ventricle

 L. _____ Tricuspid (right AV) valve

 M. _____ Venae cavae

9. Name the three layers of the heart wall.

 A._____

 B._____

 C._____

10. Name the four cardiac valves and describe their locations.

 A._____
 _____

 B._____
 _____

 C._____
 _____

 D._____
 _____

11. Define cardiac output. _____
 _____
 _____
 _____

12. What is the function of the bundle of His?
 _____
 _____
 _____
 _____

13. Name and describe the two layers of the pleura.

 A._____
 _____

 B._____
 _____

14. What structures are contained within the mediastinum? _____
 _____
 _____
 _____

15. Name the principal muscles of inspiration.

    A. _____

    B. _____

■ Exercise B – Pathology

1. List three methods used to detect lung tumors.

    A. _____

    B. _____

    C. _____

2. Describe the condition known as flail chest.

    _____

    _____

    _____

    _____

3. Penetrating chest trauma will result in which condition? What treatment is necessary?_____

    _____

    _____

    _____

    _____

4. What is cardiac tamponade? What treatment is necessary? _____

    _____

    _____

    _____

    _____

5. List the three types of thoracic outlet syndrome and the cause of each.

    A. _____

    _____

    B. _____

    _____

    C. _____

    _____

6. Describe a Type II dissecting aneurysm of the thoracic aorta. What does dissecting mean in reference to an aneurysm?_____

    _____

    _____

    _____

7. What is the composition of an atheroma? What causes formation of an atheroma?_____

    _____

    _____

    _____

8. Which cardiac enzyme levels rise following myocardial infarction?

    A. _____

    B. _____

    C. _____

9. List three complications of myocardial infarction.

    A. _____

    B. _____

    C. _____

10. What effect does alcohol have on cardiac tissue?

    _____

    _____

    _____

    _____

11. Describe the condition known as patent ductus arteriosus, list the symptoms, and provide treatment options._____

    _____

    _____

    _____

    _____

12. List the four cardiac defects seen in the classic form of tetralogy of Fallot.

    A. _____

    B. _____

    C. _____

    D. _____

13. List two variable and two inherited risk factors for coronary atherosclerosis.

    A. _____

    B. _____

    C. _____

    D. _____

14. What is/are the cause(s) of mitral regurgitation?

    _____

    _____

    _____

    _____

15. A commissurotomy is performed to treat which condition? _____

    _____

    _____

    _____

■ Exercise C – Operation

1. List the two types of mediastinoscopy, and provide a brief description of each.

    A. _____

    _____

    B. _____

    _____

2. Is bronchoscopy strictly a diagnostic procedure? Explain your answer. _____

    _____

    _____

    _____

3. In which position will the patient be placed in order to accomplish a posterolateral thoracotomy?

    _____

    _____

    _____

4. Explain the difference between lobectomy and pneumonectomy. _____

    _____

    _____

    _____

5. What is the purpose of inserting a double-lumen endotracheal tube during a thoracotomy?

    _____

    _____

    _____

    _____

6. In which position will the patient be placed to accomplish a median sternotomy? _____

    _____

    _____

    _____

    _____

7. What is empyema? What procedure is performed to treat empyema? _____

    _____

    _____

    _____

8. Which body functions are taken over by the pump oxygenator during open-heart surgery?

    _____

    _____

    _____

9. Describe the placement of the cannulas necessary for a cardiopulmonary bypass. _____

_____

_____

_____

_____

10. Name two blood vessels that are most commonly used as the graft during CABG procedures.

A. _____

B. _____

11. List the two basic types of materials that are used for cardiac valve replacement.

A. _____

B. _____

12. What are the two main components of a pacemaker?

A. _____

B. _____

13. Why is it important to have an open-heart team on "standby" during PTCA? _____

_____

_____

_____

_____

14. Is cardiopulmonary bypass necessary for closure of a patent ductus arteriosus in an infant?

_____

_____

_____

_____

15. What is the purpose of administering potassium cardioplegia solution during open-heart procedures? __

_____

_____

_____

_____

■ Exercise D – Specific Variations

Student Name _____ Date _____

Instructor _____

Surgical Procedure – Student Case Study Report

The student will be provided with basic patient information (real or simulated) and is expected to complete
the following case study.

1. Procedure name: _____
   _____
   _____

2. Definition of procedure: _____
   _____
   _____
   _____

3. What is the purpose of the procedure?_____
   _____
   _____
   _____
   _____

4. What is the expected outcome of the procedure?
   _____
   _____
   _____

5. Patient age:_____

6. Gender:_____

7. Additional pertinent patient information: _____
   _____
   _____
   _____

8. Probable preoperative diagnosis: _____
   _____
   _____
   _____
   _____

9. How was the diagnosis determined? _____
   _____
   _____
   _____
   _____

10. Discuss the relevant anatomy. _____
    _____
    _____
    _____
    _____

11. List the general and procedure-specific equipment
    that will be needed for the procedure.
    _____   _____
    _____   _____
    _____   _____
    _____   _____
    _____   _____
    _____   _____

12. List the general and procedure-specific instruments that will be needed for the procedure.

_____   _____

_____   _____

_____   _____

_____   _____

_____   _____

_____   _____

13. List the basic and procedure-specific supplies that will be needed for the procedure.

Pack _____

Basin _____

Gloves _____

Blades _____

Drapes _____

_____

Drains _____

Dressings _____

_____

Suture—Type of Suture, Needle (if applicable), and Anticipated Tissue Usage

_____   _____

_____   _____

_____   _____

_____   _____

_____   _____

_____   _____

Pharmaceuticals

_____   _____

_____   _____

_____   _____

_____   _____

Miscellaneous

_____   _____

_____   _____

_____   _____

_____   _____

_____   _____

_____   _____

14. Operative preparation: _____

_____

_____

_____

_____

_____

_____

15. What type of anesthesia will likely be used? Why?

_____

_____

_____

_____

_____

16. List any special anesthesia equipment that may be needed. _____

_____

_____

_____

_____

_____

17. Patient position during the procedure: _____

_____

_____

_____

18. What supplies will be necessary for positioning?

_____

_____

_____

_____

19. What type of shave/skin preparation will be necessary (if any)?_____

_____

_____

_____

_____

20. Define the anatomic perimeters of the prep.

_____

_____

_____

_____

_____

21. List the order in which the drapes will be applied, and describe any specific variations.

_____

_____

_____

_____

_____

22. List any practical considerations.

_____

_____

_____

_____

_____

23. List the procedural steps, and describe the preparatory and supportive actions of the STSR during each step (use additional space if necessary).

Operative Procedure	Technical Considerations
1.	•
	•
2.	•
	•
3.	•
	•
4.	•
	•
5.	•
	•
6.	•
	•

Operative Procedure (continued)	**Technical Considerations** (continued)
7.	•
	•
8.	•
	•
9.	•
	•
10.	•
	•

24. What is the postoperative diagnosis? _____

_____

_____

_____

_____

_____

25. Describe the immediate postoperative care.

_____

_____

_____

_____

_____

26. What is the patient's long-term prognosis?

_____

_____

_____

_____

_____

_____

27. What are the possible complications? _____

_____

_____

_____

_____

_____

_____

28. Comments or questions: _____

_____

_____

_____

_____

_____

29. What is the most valuable information you obtained from preparing this surgical procedure case study?

_____

_____

_____

_____

■ **Case Studies**

☐ CASE STUDY 1

Elroy has been transported to the emergency department following a motor vehicle accident (MVA). He was the unrestrained driver of one of the vehicles, and his body hit the steering wheel on impact. Elroy has dyspnea, tachypnea, and tachycardia, appears extremely anxious, and is showing signs of shock. Upon examination, the emergency physician notes distant heart sounds, hypotension, and jugular venous distension. A Swan-Ganz catheter placed by the physician reveals equal RA and pulmonary capillary wedge pressures and an elevated CVP.

1. What type of injury is suspected as a result of the blunt chest trauma? _____

_____

_____

_____

_____

2. What diagnostic exams are indicated? _____

_____

_____

_____

_____

3. What is the treatment for this condition? _____

_____

_____

_____

_____

☐

☐ CASE STUDY 2

Timothy, a 49-year-old construction worker, fell from a scaffold and was rushed to the emergency department, where he was evaluated by the trauma team. Timothy complained of chest pain, and severe respiratory distress was noted by the physician. Chest X-ray revealed fractures of the fifth and sixth ribs on the right and absence of lung markings over the affected area.

1. In addition to Timothy's fractured ribs, what other condition is affecting him? _____

_____

_____

_____

_____

2. What treatment will be provided? _____

_____

_____

_____

_____

3. What type of wound drainage system will be needed? Why? _____

_____

_____

_____

_____

4. Will a wound dressing be necessary? If so, what type and why? _____

_____

_____

_____

_____

☐

CHAPTER 23

Peripheral Vascular Surgery

OBJECTIVES

After studying this chapter, the reader should be able to:

A 1. Discuss the relevant anatomy of the peripheral vascular system.

P 2. Describe the pathology that prompts surgical intervention of the peripheral vascular system and the related terminology.

3. Discuss any special preoperative peripheral vascular diagnostic procedures.

O 4. Discuss any special preoperative preparation procedures.

5. Identify the names and uses of peripheral vascular instruments, supplies, and drugs.

6. Identify the names and uses of special equipment.

7. Discuss the intraoperative preparation of the patient undergoing the peripheral vascular procedure.

8. Define and give an overview of the peripheral vascular procedure.

9. Discuss the purpose and expected outcomes of the peripheral vascular procedure.

10. Discuss the immediate postoperative care and possible complications of the peripheral vascular procedure.

S 11. Discuss any specific variations related to the preoperative, intraoperative, and postoperative care of the patient undergoing peripheral vascular surgery.

■ Select Key Terms

Define the following:

1. adventitia _____

_____

2. bifurcation _____

_____

3. capillary _____

_____

4. claudication _____

_____

5. contralateral _____

_____

6. diastole _____

_____

7. embolus _____

_____

8. Fogarty catheter _____

_____

9. in situ _____

_____

10. innominate _____

_____

11. intima _____

_____

12. ischemia _____

_____

13. mitigate _____

_____

14. morbidity _____

_____

15. mortality _____

_____

16. occlusion _____

_____

17. papaverine _____

_____

18. patency _____

_____

19. phrenic _____

_____

20. pledget _____

_____

21. plethysmography _____

_____

22. sinus _____

_____

23. thrombus _____

_____

24. valve _____

_____

■ Exercise A – Anatomy

1. Identify the branches of the aorta shown in Figure 23-1.

   A. _____

   B. _____

   C. _____

   D. _____

   E. _____

   F. _____

   G. _____

   H. _____

   I. _____

   J. _____

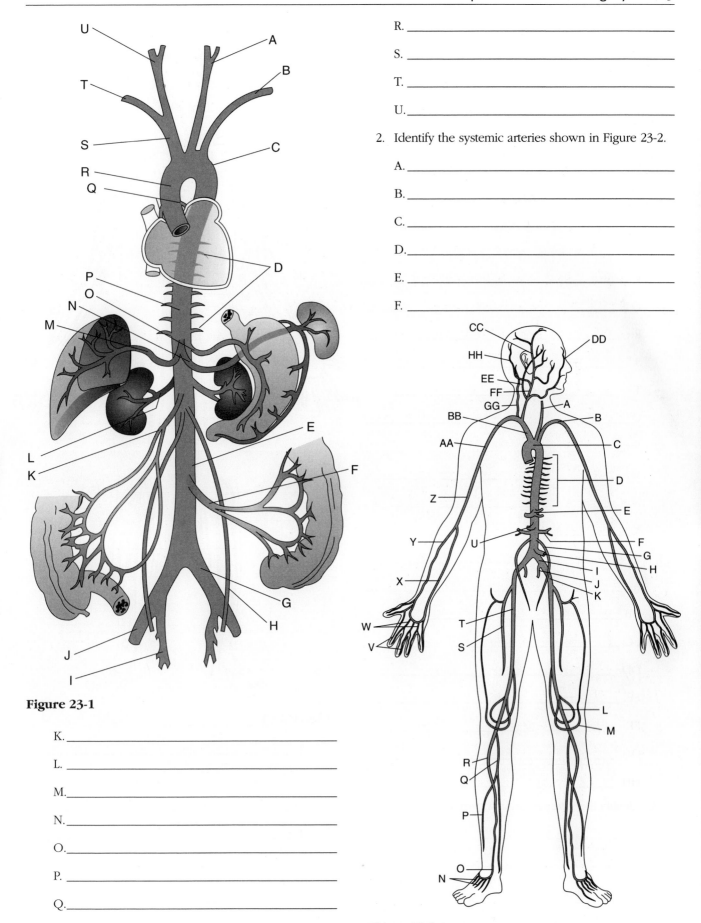

Figure 23-1

Figure 23-2

R. _____

S. _____

T. _____

U. _____

2. Identify the systemic arteries shown in Figure 23-2.

A. _____

B. _____

C. _____

D. _____

E. _____

F. _____

K. _____

L. _____

M. _____

N. _____

O. _____

P. _____

Q. _____

G._____

H._____

I._____

J._____

K._____

L._____

M._____

N._____

O._____

P._____

Q._____

R._____

S._____

T._____

U._____

V._____

W._____

X._____

Y._____

Z._____

AA._____

BB._____

CC._____

DD._____

EE._____

FF._____

GG._____

HH._____

3. Identify the systemic veins shown in Figure 23-3.

A._____

B._____

C._____

D._____

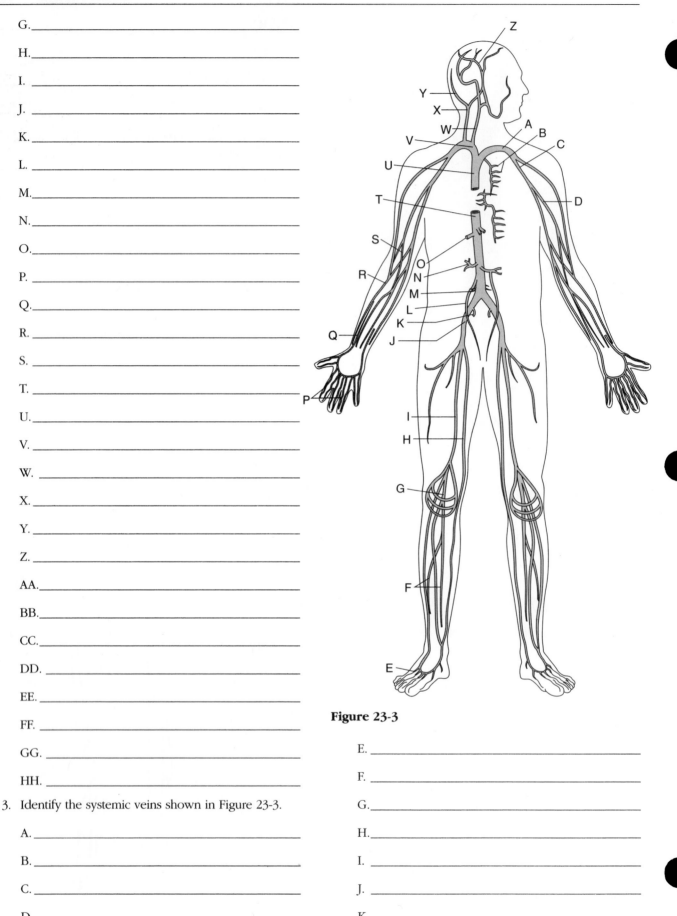

Figure 23-3

E._____

F._____

G._____

H._____

I._____

J._____

K._____

L. _____

M. _____

N. _____

O. _____

P. _____

Q. _____

R. _____

S. _____

T. _____

U. _____

V. _____

W. _____

X. _____

Y. _____

Z. _____

4. Identify the structures of the blood vessels shown in Figure 23-4.

A. _____

B. _____

C. _____

D. _____

E. _____

F. _____

G. _____

H. _____

I. _____

5. List the three tunics of a blood vessel wall, and briefly describe the composition and function of each structure.

A. _____

_____

B. _____

_____

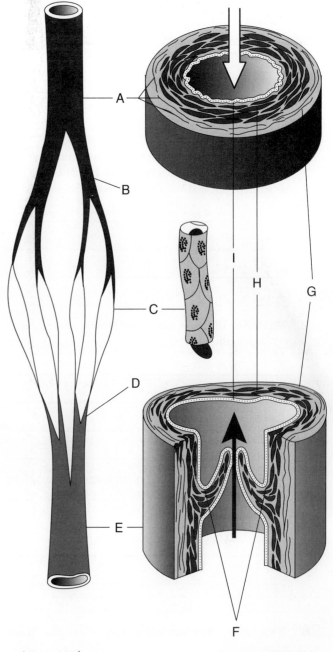

Figure 23-4

C. _____

_____

6. What structures receive arterial blood from the brachiocephalic artery? _____

_____

_____

_____

7. Which artery or arteries, if any, branch off the ascending aorta? _____

_____

_____

_____

_____

8. Each common carotid artery bifurcates into two sections. Provide the names of the two branches and the structures supplied with arterial blood from each.

A. _____

_____

B. _____

_____

9. What effect does the autonomic nervous system have on vasoconstriction? _____

_____

_____

_____

_____

10. Which is larger, the lumen of an artery or the lumen of a vein in a similar location? _____

_____

_____

_____

_____

11. What effect does vasodilation have on the blood pressure? _____

_____

_____

_____

_____

12. What is blood pressure? _____

_____

_____

_____

_____

13. List three factors that affect arterial blood pressure.

A. _____

B. _____

C. _____

14. What does the term *resistance* describe within the cardiovascular system? How does increased resistance affect blood pressure? _____

_____

_____

_____

_____

15. List the three main branches of the common hepatic artery, and name the structure(s) served by each.

A. _____

_____

B. _____

_____

C. _____

_____

■ Exercise B – Pathology

1. What causes claudication? _____

_____

_____

_____

_____

2. List the four signs/symptoms of acute arterial occlusion.

A. _____

B. _____

C. _____

D. _____

3. There are several types of emboli. Name two.

A. _____

B. _____

4. List three types of treatment for embolism.

   A. _____

   B. _____

   C. _____

5. What is the shape of a fusiform aneurysm? What portion of the aorta is most often involved?

   _____

   _____

   _____

   _____

6. Varicose veins commonly involve the saphenous vein. Describe the condition, and list two possible treatments. _____

   _____

   _____

   _____

7. What term is used to describe inflammation of a vein?

   _____

   _____

   _____

   _____

8. What is the cause of a TIA (transient ischemic attack)?

   _____

   _____

   _____

   _____

9. What is plaque? _____

   _____

   _____

   _____

   _____

10. What examinations may be performed to identify a lesion of the common carotid artery?

    _____

    _____

    _____

    _____

11. What is the difference between ischemia and necrosis? _____

    _____

    _____

    _____

    _____

    _____

12. What are the signs/symptoms associated with a TIA?

    _____

    _____

    _____

    _____

    _____

13. List four risk factors associated with the development of peripheral vascular disease.

    A. _____

    B. _____

    C. _____

    D. _____

14. How is the establishment of collateral blood flow encouraged in patients with vascular insufficiency of the lower extremity? _____

    _____

    _____

    _____

    _____

15. List three physical signs of vascular insufficiency of the lower extremity.

    A. _____

    B. _____

    C. _____

■ Exercise C – Operation

1. In what situation will contrast solution (e.g., Conray, Hypaque) be needed on the sterile field?

    _____

    _____

    _____

    _____

2. List three hemostatic agents that are typically used during peripheral vascular surgical procedures.

    A. _____

    B. _____

    C. _____

3. What is a Fogarty catheter used to accomplish?

    _____

    _____

    _____

    _____

4. What is the purpose of an intraluminal stent?

    _____

    _____

    _____

    _____

5. Vascular grafts are available in several configurations. Name two.

    A. _____

    B. _____

6. Why do some types of vascular graft material have rigid rings (exoskeleton) built into the graft? In which location are the reinforced grafts commonly implanted?_____

    _____

    _____

7. What is the primary indication for carotid endarterectomy? _____

    _____

    _____

    _____

    _____

8. During carotid endarterectomy, is the use of a shunt necessary? Why?_____

    _____

    _____

    _____

    _____

9. Vascular grafts are available in several materials. Name two.

    A. _____

    B. _____

10. What instruments are typically used to perform an arteriotomy? _____

    _____

    _____

    _____

11. What is the purpose of creating a tunnel during a femoral popliteal bypass? _____

    _____

    _____

    _____

12. List two complications that may arise following implantation of a composite graft.

    A. _____

    B. _____

13. Why is it necessary to pre-clot a vascular graft that is made of knitted polyester? _____

    _____

    _____

    _____

    _____

14. What is a patch suture? How is it prepared?

    _____

    _____

    _____

    _____

15. Why is it important for the STSR to remain sterile and keep the back table and Mayo stand intact until the patient has been transported to the PACU? _____

    _____

    _____

    _____

    _____

    _____

    _____

■ Exercise D – Specific Variations

Student Name _____ Date _____

Instructor _____

Surgical Procedure – Student Case Study Report

The student will be provided with basic patient information (real or simulated) and is expected to complete the following case study.

1. Procedure name: _____

   _____

   _____

2. Definition of procedure: _____

   _____

   _____

   _____

3. What is the purpose of the procedure? _____

   _____

   _____

   _____

   _____

4. What is the expected outcome of the procedure?

   _____

   _____

   _____

   _____

5. Patient age: _____

6. Gender: _____

7. Additional pertinent patient information: _____

   _____

   _____

   _____

8. Probable preoperative diagnosis: _____

   _____

   _____

   _____

   _____

   _____

   _____

9. How was the diagnosis determined? _____

   _____

   _____

   _____

   _____

10. Discuss the relevant anatomy. _____

    _____

    _____

    _____

    _____

    _____

    _____

11. List the general and procedure-specific equipment that will be needed for the procedure.

    _____   _____

    _____   _____

    _____   _____

    _____   _____

    _____   _____

12. List the general and procedure-specific instruments that will be needed for the procedure.

_____   _____

_____   _____

_____   _____

_____   _____

_____   _____

_____   _____

13. List the basic and procedure-specific supplies that will be needed for the procedure.

Pack _____

Basin _____

Gloves _____

Blades _____

Drapes _____

_____

Drains _____

Dressings _____

_____

Suture—Type of Suture, Needle (if applicable), and Anticipated Tissue Usage

_____   _____

_____   _____

_____   _____

_____   _____

_____   _____

Pharmaceuticals

_____   _____

_____   _____

_____   _____

_____   _____

Miscellaneous

_____   _____

_____   _____

_____   _____

_____   _____

_____   _____

_____   _____

14. Operative preparation: _____

_____

_____

_____

_____

_____

15. What type of anesthesia will likely be used? Why?

_____

_____

_____

_____

16. List any special anesthesia equipment that may be needed. _____

_____

_____

_____

_____

_____

17. Patient position during the procedure: _____

_____

_____

_____

18. What supplies will be necessary for positioning?

_____

_____

_____

_____

19. What type of shave/skin preparation will be necessary (if any)?_____

_____

_____

_____

20. Define the anatomic perimeters of the prep.

_____

_____

_____

_____

21. List the order in which the drapes will be applied, and describe any specific variations._____

_____

_____

_____

_____

_____

_____

22. List any practical considerations. _____

_____

_____

_____

_____

23. List the procedural steps, and describe the preparatory and supportive actions of the STSR during each step (use additional space if necessary).

Operative Procedure	Technical Considerations
1.	•
	•
2.	•
	•
3.	•
	•
4.	•
	•
5.	•
	•
6.	•
	•

Operative Procedure *(continued)*	**Technical Considerations** *(continued)*
7.	•
	•
8.	•
	•
9.	•
	•
10.	•
	•

24. What is the postoperative diagnosis? _____

_____

_____

_____

_____

25. Describe the immediate postoperative care.

_____

_____

_____

_____

26. What is the patient's long-term prognosis?

_____

_____

_____

_____

27. What are the possible complications? _____

_____

_____

_____

_____

_____

_____

28. Comments or questions: _____

_____

_____

_____

_____

_____

29. What is the most valuable information you obtained from preparing this surgical procedure case study?

_____

_____

_____

_____

■ **Case Studies**

☐ CASE STUDY 1

Joe is a 50-year-old male who was brought to the emergency department in hemorrhagic shock due to a ruptured abdominal aneurysm. The surgeon called the surgery department to alert them that he is in tran- sit with the patient for immediate intervention. The OR team leader, in turn, has notified the STSR and cir- culator who are assigned to the case. The surgical team springs into action.

1. What supplies will the STSR open onto the sterile field first? _____

_____

_____

_____

_____

2. What instrument sets will be needed? _____

_____

_____

_____

_____

3. What instruments will be needed first? _____

_____

_____

_____

_____

☐

☐ CASE STUDY 2

Wayne, a 67-year-old male, presented to the emergency department with the following symptoms: severe hypertension, malaise, orthopnea, peripheral edema, and decreased urinary output. He is a pack-a-day smoker and is grossly overweight.

1. What is the preliminary diagnosis? _____

    _____

    _____

    _____

    _____

2. What diagnostic examination is considered the gold standard for confirmation of the preliminary diagnosis?

    _____

    _____

    _____

    _____

3. Will surgical intervention be necessary? If so, what procedure will be scheduled? _____

    _____

    _____

    _____

    _____

24

OBJECTIVES

After studying this chapter, the reader should be able to:

A
P   1. Discuss the relevant anatomy and physiology of the neurological system.

2. Describe the pathology that prompts surgical intervention of the neurological system and the related terminology.

3. Discuss any special preoperative neurological diagnostic procedures/tests.

O   4. Discuss any special preoperative preparation procedures related to neurosurgery.

5. Identify the names and uses of neurosurgical instruments, supplies, and drugs.

6. Identify the names and uses of special equipment related to neurosurgery.

7. Discuss the intraoperative preparation of the patient undergoing the neurosurgical procedure.

8. Define and give an overview of the neurosurgical procedure.

9. Discuss the purpose and expected outcomes of the neurosurgical procedure.

10. Discuss the immediate postoperative care and possible complications of the neurosurgical procedure.

S   11. Discuss any specific variations related to the preoperative, intraoperative, and postoperative care of the neurosurgical patient.

12. Discuss recent advances in neurosurgery.

■ Select Key Terms

Define the following:

1. abscess _____

_____

2. acute _____

_____

3. autonomic nervous system _____

_____

4. cerebellum _____

_____

5. cerebrum _____

_____

6. circle of Willis _____

_____

7. CNS _____

_____

8. decompress _____

_____

9. dysraphism _____

_____

10. epidural _____

_____

11. extruded _____

_____

12. glioma _____

_____

13. hematoma _____

_____

14. ICP _____

_____

15. integration _____

_____

16. meninges _____

_____

17. osteophyte _____

_____

18. parasympathetic nervous system _____

_____

19. PNS _____

_____

20. radiculopathy _____

_____

21. somatic nervous system _____

_____

22. sympathetic nervous system _____

_____

23. TIA _____

_____

24. transphenoidal _____

_____

■ **Exercise A – Anatomy**

1. Identify the major divisions of the autonomic nervous system shown in Figure 24-1.

    A. _____

    B. _____

    C. _____

    D. _____

    E. _____

F. _____

G. _____

H. _____

I. _____

J. _____

K. _____

2. Identify the structures of the external surface of the brain shown in Figure 24-2.

    A. _____

    B. _____

    C. _____

    D. _____

    E. _____

    F. _____

    G. _____

    H. _____

    I. _____

    J. _____

    K. _____

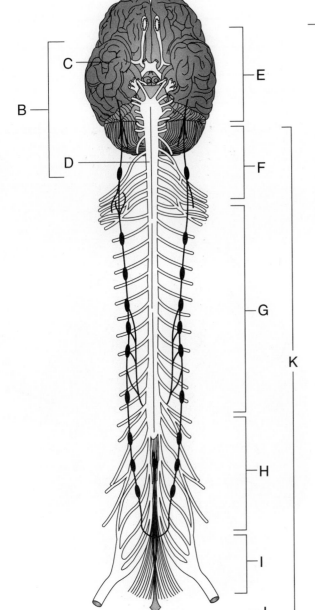

Figure 24-1

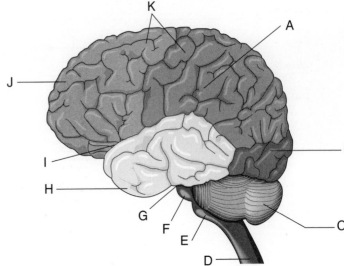

Figure 24-2

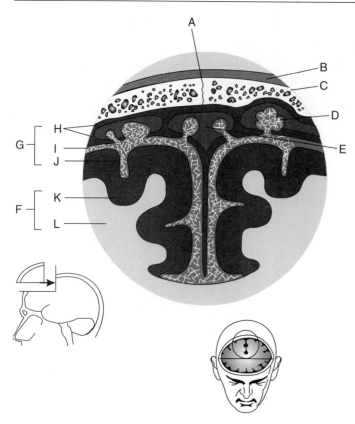

Figure 24-3

4. Identify the cranial nerves shown in Figure 24-4.

A. _____

B. _____

C. _____

D. _____

E. _____

F. _____

G. _____

H. _____

I. _____

J. _____

K. _____

L. _____

M. _____

3. Identify the meninges and related structures shown in Figure 24-3.

A. _____

B. _____

C. _____

D. _____

E. _____

F. _____

G. _____

H. _____

I. _____

J. _____

K. _____

L. _____

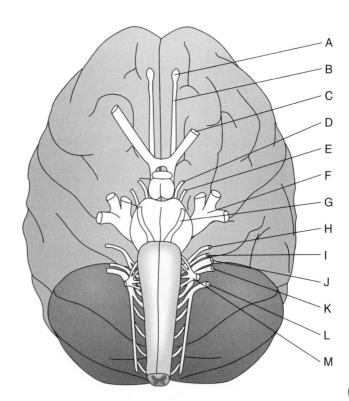

Figure 24-4

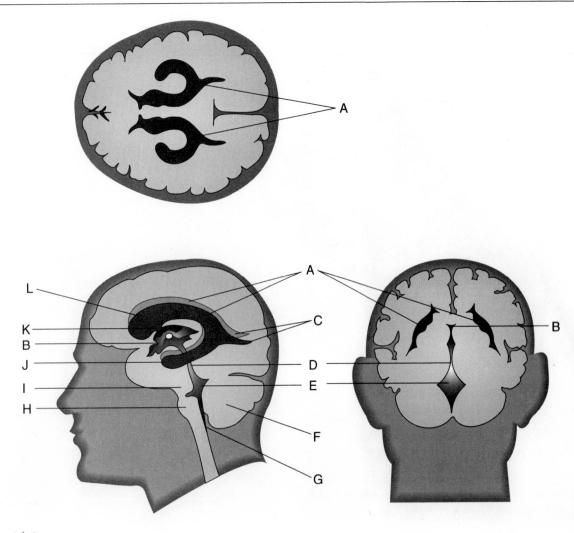

Figure 24-5

5. Identify the ventricles of the brain and related structures shown in Figure 24-5.

A. _____

B. _____

C. _____

D. _____

E. _____

F. _____

G. _____

H. _____

I. _____

J. _____

K. _____

L. _____

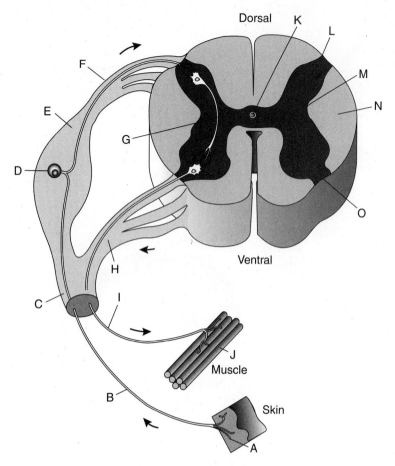

Dorsal

Ventral

Muscle

Skin

Figure 24-6

6. Identify the pathway of impulses (reflex arc) and related structures shown in Figure 24-6.

   A. _____

   B. _____

   C. _____

   D. _____

   E. _____

   F. _____

   G. _____

   H. _____

   I. _____

   J. _____

   K. _____

   L. _____

   M. _____

   N. _____

   O. _____

7. Name the eight bones of the cranium.

   A. _____

   B. _____

   C. _____

   D. _____

   E. _____

   F. _____

   G. _____

   H. _____

8. Name the three meningeal layers in sequence from
   outermost to innermost.

   A. _____

   B. _____

   C. _____

9. Where is CSF formed? How is it formed? _____

_____

_____

_____

10. Name the three branches of the trigeminal nerve, and describe the functions of the target tissue(s) innervated by each branch.

A. _____

_____

B. _____

_____

C. _____

_____

11. What are the three primary functions of the nervous system?

A. _____

_____

B. _____

_____

C. _____

_____

12. What are the two subdivisions of the ANS, and what is the basic function of each division?

A. _____

_____

B. _____

_____

13. What is the circle of Willis? _____

_____

_____

_____

14. The auditory processing area of the brain is located in the _____ lobe of the brain.

15. The vital centers of the brain (respiratory, cardiac, vasomotor) are contained in which portion of the brain stem? _____

_____

_____

_____

■ Exercise B – Pathology

1. Hydrocephalus has several causes. List three.

A. _____

B. _____

C. _____

2. List three types of obstruction of the aqueduct between the ventricles that can lead to hydrocephalus.

A. _____

B. _____

C. _____

3. Describe the condition known as spondylosis.

_____

_____

_____

_____

_____

4. Name two radiographic techniques that may be used to identify spinal disorders, and describe how each is used.

A. _____

_____

B. _____

_____

5. What is the difference between a subdural hematoma and an epidural hematoma? _____

_____

_____

_____

6. Define craniosynostosis, and describe the method(s) for diagnosing the condition. _____

_____

_____

_____

7. Describe spina bifida. _____

_____

_____

_____

8. List the three classifications (locations) of spinal cord tumors and the symptoms of each.

A. _____

_____

B. _____

_____

C. _____

_____

9. Carpal tunnel syndrome affects which nerve at what level? _____

_____

_____

_____

10. What is the underlying cause of growth hormone (GH) overproduction? _____

_____

_____

_____

11. Describe two symptoms that a patient with herniated nucleus pulposus may experience.

A. _____

B. _____

12. What is the most common type of brain tumor?

_____

_____

_____

_____

13. What symptoms are associated with acoustic neuroma? Which nerve is affected? _____

_____

_____

_____

14. The condition known as tic douloureux is also known as _____ _____ . What surgical procedure is performed to relieve the symptoms of tic douloureux? _____

_____

_____

_____

15. List and describe the three types of subdural hematoma.

A. _____

_____

B. _____

_____

C. _____

_____

■ Exercise C – Operation

1. What is the Mayfield pin-fixation device used to accomplish? _____

_____

_____

_____

2. How do Raney clips differ from aneurysm clips?

_____

_____

_____

_____

3. Access to the occipital lobe of the brain may be accomplished with the patient in either of two positions. Name the two possible positions.

   A. _____

   B. _____

4. What supplies may be necessary to remove scalp hair in the operating room? _____

_____

_____

_____

5. List three options for treatment of a cerebral aneurysm.

   A. _____

   B. _____

   C. _____

6. It is important to restrict movement in and around the sterile field at all times, but why is this especially true during procedures near the cerebellopontine angle?

_____

_____

_____

_____

7. List the four main components of the ventriculoperitoneal shunt.

   A. _____

   B. _____

   C. _____

   D. _____

8. Name two approaches that can be used for surgery of the pituitary.

   A. _____

   B. _____

9. List two materials that can be implanted during cranioplasty and that can be molded to fit the cranial defect.

   A. _____

   B. _____

10. List two methods by which the bone flap is secured to the cranium following a craniotomy.

   A. _____

   B. _____

11. Why are two separate Mayo stands needed for transphenoidal procedures? _____

_____

_____

_____

_____

12. What is papaverine used for during arterial intracranial surgery? _____

_____

_____

_____

_____

13. What is the ideal temperature for irrigation fluid that will be used intracranially? _____

_____

_____

_____

14. What is the CUSA, and how is it used?

_____

_____

_____

_____

15. What is ICP? How is it monitored?

_____

_____

_____

_____

■ **Exercise D – Specific Variations**

Student Name _____ Date _____

Instructor _____

The student will be provided with basic patient information (real or simulated) and is expected to complete the following case study.

1. Procedure name: _____

   _____

   _____

2. Definition of procedure: _____

   _____

   _____

   _____

3. What is the purpose of the procedure? _____

   _____

   _____

   _____

   _____

4. What is the expected outcome of the procedure?

   _____

   _____

   _____

   _____

5. Patient age: _____

6. Gender: _____

7. Additional pertinent patient information: _____

   _____

   _____

   _____

8. Probable preoperative diagnosis: _____

   _____

   _____

   _____

   _____

9. How was the diagnosis determined? _____

   _____

   _____

   _____

10. Discuss the relevant anatomy. _____

    _____

    _____

    _____

    _____

    _____

11. List the general and procedure-specific equipment that will be needed for the procedure.

    _____   _____

    _____   _____

    _____   _____

    _____   _____

    _____   _____

    _____   _____

12. List the general and procedure-specific instruments that will be needed for the procedure.

_____   _____

_____   _____

_____   _____

_____   _____

_____   _____

_____   _____

13. List the basic and procedure-specific supplies that will be needed for the procedure.

Pack _____

Basin _____

Gloves _____

Blades _____

Drapes _____

_____

Drains _____

Dressings _____

_____

Suture—Type of Suture, Needle (if applicable), and Anticipated Tissue Usage

_____   _____

_____   _____

_____   _____

_____   _____

_____   _____

Pharmaceuticals

_____   _____

_____   _____

_____   _____

_____   _____

_____   _____

Miscellaneous

_____   _____

_____   _____

_____   _____

_____   _____

_____   _____

14. Operative preparation: _____

_____

_____

_____

_____

15. What type of anesthesia will likely be used? Why?

_____

_____

_____

_____

_____

16. List any special anesthesia equipment that may be needed. _____

_____

_____

_____

_____

17. Patient position during the procedure: _____

_____

_____

_____

18. What supplies will be necessary for positioning?

_____

_____

_____

_____

19. What type of shave/skin preparation will be necessary (if any)?_____

_____

_____

_____

_____

20. Define the anatomic perimeters of the prep.

_____

_____

_____

_____

21. List the order in which the drapes will be applied, and describe any specific variations.

_____

_____

_____

_____

_____

_____

_____

22. List any practical considerations.

_____

_____

_____

_____

_____

23. List the procedural steps, and describe the preparatory and supportive actions of the STSR during each step (use additional space if necessary).

Operative Procedure	Technical Considerations
1.	•
	•
2.	•
	•
3.	•
	•
4.	•
	•
5.	•
	•

(continues)

Operative Procedure *(continued)*	Technical Considerations *(continued)*
6.	•
	•
7.	•
	•
8.	•
	•
9.	•
	•
10.	•
	•

24. What is the postoperative diagnosis? _____

_____

_____

_____

_____

_____

25. Describe the immediate postoperative care.

_____

_____

_____

_____

_____

_____

26. What is the patient's long-term prognosis?

_____

_____

_____

_____

_____

_____

27. What are the possible complications? _____

_____

_____

_____

_____

_____

_____

28. Comments or questions: _____

_____

_____

_____

_____

_____

29. What is the most valuable information you obtained from preparing this surgical procedure case study?

_____

_____

_____

_____